MEDICINAL POWER OF CANNABIS

MEDICINAL POWER OF CANNABIS

Using a Natural Herb to Heal Arthritis,
Nausea, Pain, and Other Ailments

JOHN HICKS

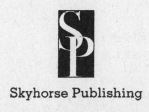

Skyhorse Publishing

Skyhorse Publishing books may be purchased in bulk at special discounts for sales promotion, corporate gifts, fund-raising, or educational purposes. Special editions can also be created to specifications. For details, contact the Special Sales Department, Skyhorse Publishing, 307 West 36th Street, 11th Floor, New York, NY 10018 or info@skyhorsepublishing.com.

Skyhorse® and Skyhorse Publishing® are registered trademarks of Skyhorse Publishing, Inc.®, a Delaware corporation.

Visit our website at www.skyhorsepublishing.com.

10 9 8 7 6 5

Library of Congress Cataloging-in-Publication Data is available on file.

Cover design by Rain Saukas
Cover art credit i-Stock

Print ISBN: 978-1-63450-583-3
Ebook ISBN: 978-1-63450-873-5

Printed in the United States of America

Contents

Acknowledgements

A heartfelt thank you to my beautiful wife Betsy. Your support and understanding were beyond expectation. I appreciate your willingness to be without a kitchen table for 18 months, as it was covered in papers, journals, and books while I researched and wrote.

I also wish to thank Elizabeth Aquino for her hard work and dedication to helping me to express myself.

A special thank you to Dr. Marcey Shapiro, who gave me insight into the use of medicinal herbs, including cannabis, and to Teri Arranga for her encouragement and support to write this book.

Thank you, and love to you all!

John

I

History of Hemp

Hemp, from the plant *cannabis sativa*, and its sister plants, *cannabis indica* and *cannabis ruderalis*, has a rich and varied history of use, including hemp fibers for textiles, the oil, the seeds for medicine and, of course, the plant itself for psychotropic activity. Although the exact date of its first use is unknown, records and artifacts indicate that hemp has been cultivated for more than 10,000 years.

We know that hemp has been cultivated in China since 4000 BCE. The first identified paper, in China around 1000 BCE, was made from hemp. It was very white and extremely durable, lasting for long periods of time without decomposing.[1] Hemp cords in pottery from Mesopotamia date back over 10,000 years, and fabrics made with hemp have been dated to 8000 BCE in what is now modern Taiwan, as well as textiles found in China and Turkestan dated around 4000 BCE. In the book *The Natural History*, Pliny the Elder describes the use of hemp rope, and of marijuana providing analgesic effects. In the years between 2000 and 800 BCE, the plant was recorded in the Hindu sacred text Athuruveda as sacred grass; it was considered one of the five sacred plants in India, used both medicinally and for rituals and ceremonies. Psychotropic properties were first described between 100 BCE and 1 CE, reported by Chinese herbalist Pen Tsao Ching. In 600 BCE, the Zend-Avesta, the sacred book of

Zoroastrianism, spoke of hemp's intoxicating resin being used by the people of India.

Thousands of years later, between 1606 and 1632 AD, the French and British cultivated cannabis for hemp in their colonies at Port Royal, Acadia (present-day Nova Scotia). In 1611, the British began growing it in Virginia, and by 1632 it was also grown in Plymouth, Massachusetts.[4] Hemp was used to make rope and sails for shipping and navy fleets. The colonies passed laws to encourage the production of hemp, as it was also needed for cordage and cloth. In the 1630s in Hartford, Connecticut, the colonists passed a resolution requiring every family to plant hemp.

During the 1700s, the American colonists were forbidden to weave with hemp, which kept them tied to England to purchase woven products. New England, Virginia, Pennsylvania, New York, New Jersey, and North and South Carolina were paid subsidies to grow hemp, or they were given tax credits to do so. Hemp was also used as money.[2,4] The weaving restrictions ended when Irish weavers settled in the colonies and taught the colonists their trade, beginning the production of hemp fabrics there.[184] Decades later, during World War II, hemp was grown to provide needed rope for the United States Navy. The loss of the Philippines and their Manila hemp was met by renewed US efforts to produce hemp, and the US Department of Agriculture (USDA) produced films to stimulate its production for war use. Farmers and their sons who grew hemp from 1942–1945 were waived from serving in the military.[3] Hemp was used for clothing, military uniforms, ships' rigging, shoes, parachute webbing, baggage and more.[3] In 1943, during World War II's Hemp for Victory campaign, production grew from approximately 2,000 acres to about 146,200 acres.[3]

Thousands of years after the Chinese made paper from it, cannabis hemp was used as legal tender (money) in most of the Americas between 1631 until the early 1800s.[1] Benjamin

Franklin started one of America's first paper mills with cannabis,[3,4] and both George Washington and Thomas Jefferson grew cannabis on their plantations.[3,4] Jefferson drafted both the Declaration of Independence and the Constitution of the United States on hemp paper.[3,4] In Europe, artists Rembrandt and Van Gogh painted on canvas made of hemp.

In 1916, the chief scientists of the USDA, Jason L. Merrill and Lester H. Dewey, created paper from hemp pulp, showing that it was environmentally better than wood pulp and would reduce the need for deforestation as well as the toxic chemicals released into the environment. They demonstrated that hemp pulp uses between one-seventh and one-fourth as much sulfur-based acid chemicals as wood pulp and would thereby prevent the constant release of dioxins from the production of paper. By using hemp instead of wood, hydrogen peroxide was effective as a less toxic substitute for chlorine bleach.

However, history shows us that dollars replaced common sense, and the powerful industrialists realized that the cultivation of cannabis stymied their monetary gain as long as it remained in competition with the wood-paper industry. In 1914, the Harrison Act in the United States defined the use of marijuana, among other drugs, as a crime.[6] The historical legacy is that today hemp is only legal to grow in California and Colorado and is heavily regulated; restrictions include limiting how it's grown, how the fields are fenced, lighting requirements, and the use of guards. If these restrictions were loosened, one could certainly make the case that hemp could replace wood-pulp paper, computer printout paper, corrugated boxes, and paperback books with significantly fewer adverse repercussions to the environment.

The head of the industrialists was William Randolph Hearst, who had large timber holdings that fed his paper industry and, in turn, his powerful newspaper industry. William DuPont, another influential industrialist, had a huge petrochemical industry, creating plastics, paints, and other fossil fuels. Andrew Mellon, the United States Secretary of the Treasury and owner of Gulf Oil, had a vested interest in the competitive threat of hemp cultivation and created tax breaks for the oil companies, such as the oil-depletion allowances that are still in force today. Mellon also pushed through tax plans that reduced taxes on wealthy and large corporations to encourage greater investment.

These forces combined to make hemp the object of the first "yellow" journalism.[7] To protect their interests and fortunes, these men worked with elements of government to condone and popularize movies, publications, and books about the evils of marijuana. Propaganda about marijuana had originated in Mexico, where it was banned in 1920, and found a home north of the border when Harry Anslinger, the director of the US Narcotics Bureau, began to push the theme of "reefer madness." Ainslinger, with the support of the Hearst and DuPont empires, easily convinced states to begin outlawing marijuana. He testified in Congress about the dangers of "this evil weed" in 1937, wrote editorials and letters in multiple papers, and convinced the Congress to pass the Anslinger Act. Formally known as the Marihuana Tax Act of 1937 (HR 6385), the law imposed a prohibitive tax on the importation and cultivation of hemp and hemp products and effectively criminalized marijuana use at not only state but federal level. In addition, legislation was pushed through Congress that gave tax breaks to the oil companies, to make the industrialists happy.[7]

The medical history of marijuana dates back to Emperor Chen-Nung of China,[1] who recorded the first use of cannabis as medicine in the year 2737 BCE. Those records indicate that cannabis was used to treat malaria, female disorders, and many other illnesses for more than 5,000 years. The herbalist emperor described the fruit *Ma-fen* and explained that if this fruit were taken in excess, it would produce hallucinations.[1,2] During the years between 2000 and 800 BCE, the Hindu sacred text Atharuveda referred to the plant as *sacred grass*. Considered one of the five sacred plants in India, it was used both medicinally and ritualistically in ceremonies. In 600 BCE the Zend-Avesta spoke of hemp's intoxicating resin and its use by the Indian people. Psychotropic properties of the plant and its use were first described between 100 BCE and 1 CE, reported by Chinese herbalist Pen Tsao Ching.

Between 130 and 200 AD, Greek physician Galen prescribed medical marijuana.[1] In 200, the first pharmacopeia listed medical marijuana, and on the other side of the world, the Chinese surgeon Hrea To used marijuana as an anesthetic. In 300 AD, a young woman in Jerusalem received medical marijuana to aid childbirth. On the European continent, French physicians mentioned the use of medical marijuana in 1532 AD,[1] and, in 1563, a Portuguese physician mentioned the medicinal effects of marijuana in his medical practice.[1] In 1578 China's Li Shih-Chen wrote of the antibiotic and antiemetic effects of medicinal marijuana.[1] Robert Burton, the seventeenth-century British writer, listed marijuana as a treatment for depression in his 1621 book *Anatomy of Melancholy*.[1]

More than one hundred years later, in 1764, medical marijuana appeared in New England dispensaries as a prescription option.[1] The Edinburgh New Dispensary of 1794[1] listed hemp oil as useful for coughs, venereal disease, and urinary incontinence During the 1840s in America, medicinal preparations with the cannabis base were available through this dispensary.[6] During the mid-nineteenth century, medical marijuana was used to treat rabies, rheumatism, epilepsy and tetanus; in 1842, Irish physician O'Shaughnessy published cannabis research in English medical journals.[1,2] The United States added cannabis to the pharmacopeia in 1850, and, from then until 1915, marijuana was widely used in the United States as a medicinal drug and could be easily purchased at pharmacies and general stores. In England, Sir J. R. Reynolds, chief physician to Queen Victoria, prescribed medical marijuana for her in 1890.[1]

In the United States between 1915 and 1927, cannabis began to be prohibited for nonmedical use. The government said that it had no medical benefit and could therefore no longer be used for those reasons. Industry was using imported hemp for some products and gradually replaced all US-grown hemp as the rules became too restrictive. Prior to the ban, by 1915, 8,400 acres of hemp were grown in the United States. Kentucky had 6,500 acres, and 2,000 acres were grown among Ohio, Indiana, Wisconsin, and California.[3] In 1915 California was the first state to ban cannabis, followed by Texas in 1919 and New York in 1927.

As noted earlier, in 1936, the propaganda film *Reefer Madness,* which was meant to scare American youth, was released.[306] The film depicted the dangers of marijuana consumption, vilified those who "pushed" it on unsuspecting youth, and dramatized its hallucinatory effects, with characters driven to rape, suicide, hit-and-run accidents, and even insanity. One year later, Congress passed the Marihuana Tax Act, even after Dr. William C. Woodford testified for the American Medical Association (AMA) at the congressional hearings, stating that the AMA knew of no evidence proving marijuana to be a dangerous drug. He further stated that, in effectively prohibiting its use, lawmakers were losing sight of the fact that future investigations might show that there are substantial medical uses for cannabis.[2,3] The law that was passed required a $100 transfer tax ($1,664.63 in 2014 dollars) on the sale of marijuana, making it financially prohibitive and ensuring the financial advantage to Hearst, DuPont, and Mellon.

Despite the tax, during the 1930s, Ford Motor Company saw a future for biomass fuels and operated a biomass conversion plant that used hemp. They extracted many compounds from the plant that are still used and owned by oil-related industries.[7] In 1941 Ford produced an automobile from hemp-based plastics that was both lightweight and suffered less damage when involved in a crash.[4] This automobile was also fueled by clean-burning, hemp-based methanol.[3,4] It was known that hemp oil could also produce high-grade diesel fuel, aircraft engine fuel, and high-grade machine oil, an easily renewable source of energy and clean-burning fuel. Methanol is used today in some race cars.[1]

By 1941 cannabis was removed from the *United States Pharmacopeia,* and its medical uses were no longer recognized in America.[1] The Boggs Act and the Narcotics Control Act in 1951 increased all drug penalties and laid down mandatory sentences for those convicted.[7] The National Organization for the Reform of Marijuana Laws (NORML) was formed in 1970, and, in the Comprehensive Drug Abuse Prevention and Control Act, the law replaced mandatory penalties for drug offenses for marijuana and categorized them separately from narcotics.[7]

The Shafer commission recommended that the use of cannabis be relegalized in 1972, but its recommendations were ignored.[7] Even the scientist Carl Sagan proposed that marijuana may have been the world's first agricultural crop, leading to the development of civilization itself. In 1977 he wrote that "it would be wryly interesting if in human history the cultivation of marijuana led generally to the invention of agriculture, and thereby to civilization."[5]

The drug nabilone, a cannabinoid-based medication, was released in 1975.[8] nabilone is a synthetic cannabinoid, most like delta-9-tetrahydrocannabinol (delta-9-THC), used for cancer chemotherapy-induced nausea and vomiting (CINV) and as an adjuvant for the treatment of neuropathic pain. Used in Canada, the United States, the United Kingdom and Mexico, it is produced by several companies and was FDA-approved in

1985 as dronabinol, a synthetic form of THC for cancer patients.[8] In 1986 the federal government created the Compassionate Investigational New Drug (IND) research program that allowed patients to receive up to nine pounds of cannabis from the federal government each year. Marijuana was still maintained as a Schedule 1 drug, which reflected its "high potential for abuse and no medical value." President Reagan implemented the Anti-Drug Abuse Act, which mandated minimum sentences and increased federal penalties for possession and distribution of marijuana, instituting the United States' international War on Drugs.

Despite the political climate, in 1988 the US Drug Enforcement Agency (DEA) administrative law judge Francis Young presented his findings and, after thorough hearings, found that marijuana had a clearly established medical use and recommended it be reclassified as a prescriptive drug. His recommendation was ignored.[9] The US government closed the Compassionate IND. However, in 1992, pressure mounted and dronabinol was approved for AIDS wasting syndrome.[476] Questions were raised about the pharmaceutical industry's influence and their desire to stifle competition from marijuana.

In 1996 California became the first state to really use medical marijuana, and it was legalized for people who suffer from AIDS, cancer, and other serious illnesses. This was followed by legalization in Arizona, Colorado, Maine, Montana, Nevada, Oregon, Washington, the District of Columbia, Hawaii, Maryland, New Mexico, Rhode Island, and Vermont.[7] One year later, in 1997, the American Office of National Drug Control Policy commissioned the Institute of Medicine (IOM) to do a comprehensive study of medical efficacy in cannabis therapeutics. Their conclusions were that cannabis is safe and effective, that medical patients should have access to it, and that government should expand funds for further research and drug development of marijuana. The federal government ignored these findings and refused to act on the recommendations of this study.[10] In 2001 Canada adopted federal law in support of medical marijuana, the first country in the world to approve medical marijuana nationwide.[7]

Meanwhile, in the United States, President Bill Clinton contradicted the IOM recommendations in 1997 and 2001 and continued with Reagan and George H. W. Bush's War on Drugs.[6] He continued a campaign to arrest and prosecute medical-marijuana patients and the medical providers and dispensaries in California and elsewhere. In 1999, the DEA reclassified dronabinol to a Schedule 3 drug, which made it easier to prescribe, but marijuana was still listed as a Schedule 1 drug.[516] Between 2001 and 2009, the George W. Bush administration intensified the War on Drugs, targeting both patients and doctors across the state of California.[6]

As of this writing, the entire area of marijuana and its legality is in a state of constant flux. New legislation is presently being considered to change the whole access and recommendations for the medical use of marijuana in California and other states. The California Medical Board is getting ready to change their position and rules regarding appropriate recommendations for the use of medical marijuana, but it appears that a state of flux will be ongoing.

II

Inflammation

Medications developed to control inflammation have not been effective and have many side effects. Research on marijuana shows that it works to reduce inflammation both locally and generally this is accomplished through actions on different cell types as well as effects on the immune system. We are going to see that the effects and benefits of marijuana are diverse and affect inflammation in many areas of the body, thereby helping with different diseases.

Inflammation underlies most diseases of today and needs to be modulated if we are to help control acute and chronic symptoms of disease. The word *inflammation* is derived from the Latin *inflammo,* or "to set alight." The inflammatory response is a normal one, controlled by the immune system to deal quickly and effectively with issues. Chronic inflammation ensues when the immune system is out of balance.[1] Our immune system has two sides, the TH1 side and the TH2 side. Composed of cytotoxic T cells and natural killer cells, the TH1 side helps fight viruses and fight cancer. The TH2 side of the immune system helps produce antibodies for our protection.[1, 2]

Inflammation is the response of a tissue to injury by direct trauma, irritants, toxins or pathogenic organisms such as viruses and fungi. In inflammation, blood flow increases to the tissue, as does temperature, redness, swelling, and pain. Depending on the source of the trauma, the response of tissues and the immune system will be specifically tailored to the precipitating cause.[3, 4] Pain, heat, redness, swelling, and the loss of function are the cardinal signs of inflammation.[20] Originally described by Celsus (c. 25 BCE to c. 50 CE), the original four cardinal signs were pain (*dolor*), heat (*calor*), redness (*rubor*), and swelling (*tumor*). The fifth sign, loss of function, was added by Galen in the second century CE.[21]

When the immune system is activated by bacteria, it occurs through specific bacterial surface antigens. Each bacterium has its own specific antigens. Antigens on the bacteria can also activate the complement system through the alternative pathway. Antigens, which are cell specific markers, can activate the complement system and be destroyed. When activated, the complement system helps destroy the bacteria by punching holes in the cell walls of the bacteria. Other antigens on pathogens form a pathogen-associated molecular pattern (PAMP). These antigens react with immune cells, such as leukocytes and macrophages. This iteration leads to the activation of the leukocytes through these antigens reacting with specific, toll-like receptors (TLR). The mast cells are the major tissue inhabitants from the immune system, living in the tissues and responding to the introduction of pathogens.[5, 6]

The cytoplasm of the mast cells in the tissue is loaded with granules containing mediators of inflammation. The surface of the mast cell is coated with receptors. When the proper ligand binds to the receptor, it triggers exocytosis, the release of the contents of the granules into the tissue. These cells are some of the major initiators of inflammation. The TLRs on the mast cells will trigger exocytosis when they interact with PAMPs, such as lipopolysaccharides, the endotoxins of gram-negative bacteria. Lipopolysaccharide is the endotoxin that is a normal part of the cell membrane on gram-negative bacteria. Another trigger for mast cells is the peptidoglycan of the gram-positive bacterial cell walls. Peptidoglycans react with receptors on immune cells.

Mast cells also have receptors for complement fragments that trigger exocytosis of their granules. C3a and C5a are the fragments that will trigger this reaction. Another trigger is bacteria coated with C3b fragments. Once mast cells are activated, they literally release dozens of their granules as inflammatory triggers. Some of these mediators are released immediately from the granules, while others are released later as they interact and become activated.[6]

Some of these mediators work locally to create the signs of inflammation, while others act systematically to recruit more white blood cells from the immune system to help fight the invader. The latter include monocytes, local macrophages, neutrophils, dendritic cells, and all subclasses of lymphocytes. These lymphocytes include B cells, T cells, natural killer (NK) cells, and eosinophils. Recruited cells can become activated, help fight any infection that is present, and may produce their own mediators to increase the inflammatory process. If this process continues past the point of clearing pathogens, it can create cell damage and tissue destruction. One of the most prominent mediators of inflammation is tumor necrosis factor-alpha (TNF-alpha).[7-9] TNF-alpha can quickly stimulate and turn on mast cells, which then release more TNF-alpha. When a cell is stimulated or activated by TNF-alpha through its receptors on all immune cells, it activates them quickly and they then produce large amounts of TNF-alpha, which continues the inflammatory reaction.

All immune cells involved in inflammation have receptors for TNF-alpha. This cytokine, an immune modulator, activates immune cells to produce their own cytokines and immune modulators. TNF-alpha can also induce cell differentiation and activation and lead to the progressive spread of inflammation.

TNF-alpha is only one in the family of tumor necrosis factors; these can stimulate growth of cells, produce growth inhibition, or lead to cell self-destruction (apoptosis). Specifically, TNF-alpha can lead to tumor regression, septic shock, and cachexia, a wasting syndrome. Cachexia is characterized by anorexia, net catabolism, weight loss, and anemia. Another potent mediator and cell-activity modulator is cachectin, which is equivalent to TNF-alpha. Also a potent pyrogen, TNF-alpha stimulates fever, cell proliferation, and cell differentiation.[1,10]

TNF-alpha is one of the prominent mediators seen in many and varied pathologic conditions that we presently deal with in medicine. It can induce septic shock and is one of the markers seen in cancer, AIDS, transplantation rejection, multiple sclerosis, diabetes, rheumatoid arthritis, trauma, malaria, meningitis, ischemia-reperfusion injury (the loss of blood supply and oxygen and then the reestablishment of blood flow and oxygen), and adult respiratory distress syndrome.[11] TNF-alpha induces activation and neutrophilic division during inflammation; however, if it binds to TNF-R55 receptors, cell growth is not supported and can lead to cell death. The beginning of the reaction of TNF-alpha helps to promote remodeling and replacement of injured or senescence cells, but when it persists at high levels for an extended period of time, it loses its antitumor activity.[10, 11]

TNF-alpha's ability to fight tumors is reduced for several possible reasons: It can be polymerized into chains of TNF-alpha, which are then inactive. The tumor cells can shed their TNF receptors or TNF-alpha can be broken down. Or an excessive amount of anti-TNF antibodies may be produced.[11]

Tryptase is another active compound of inflammation. The most abundant protein released by mast cells, tryptase is a protease enzyme that activates C3 of the complement system. Through this activation, the complement fractions can activate more immune cells and attack any bacteria in the vicinity. It also functions as a chemotactic cytokine and attracts more leukocytes in the area.[12]

When activated in the local area of inflammation, macrophages and neutrophils start producing reactive oxygen species (ROS). These are toxic to microorganisms and can also lead to tissue damage and the propagation of chronic inflammation.[13,14] Histamine is also contained in the granules of the mast cells and is a potent mediator released by exocytosis. Histamine works to increase blood flow to the area and causes leakage of fluid and proteins from the blood into the tissue space. The quick release and the reaction of the tissues to the histamine produce redness and swelling that is associated with inflammation.[15]

Interleukin-1 (IL-1) is found in the macrophages, monocytes, and activated platelets. This cytokine has local (paracrine) activity affecting only the cells in the local vicinity and stimulates the production of tissue factors as well as helping to trigger blood clotting cascade. IL-1 also stimulates the synthesis and secretion of other interleukins. This process helps to activate T cells and thus initiates an adaptive immune response. Interleukin also has an endocrine or hormonal effect in that it is carried through the bloodstream to the whole body. This process can lead to a reduction in blood pressure and an increase in fever. The stimulation and release of prostaglandins affect the temperature control center of the hypothalamus, causing fever production.[16]

Bradykinin is a nano-peptide (a protein fragment composed of nine amino acids) which continuously circulates in the blood. Produced in the liver, it circulates in the inactive form of a precursor called kininogen. This is one of the molecules that makes up our alpha-globulins and is activated by a proteolytic cleavage of the precursor. Bradykinin acts to relax smooth muscle and the arterioles, thereby lowering blood pressure and increasing blood flow into the tissues. It also acts to make the capillaries leaky, which then allows more blood components into the tissue space, producing redness, warmth, and some of the swelling in the inflamed tissue. Bradykinin also stimulates the release of nitric oxide and the production and release of prostaglandins.[17, 18]

Prostaglandins and leukotrienes are potent mediators of inflammation. Derived from arachiodonic acid, they are unsaturated fatty acids produced from membrane phospholipids. Cycloxygenase produces prostaglandin H2 (PGH-2) or thromboxanes, and 5-lipooxygenase will produce leukotrienes.[19] Both are powerful modulators of the inflammation process. They are active in both acute and chronic inflammation.

Acute inflammation is beneficial. It works to isolate the damage area and to mobilize protective cells and molecules to the site. This acute process works to promote the removal of damaged tissues and to increase healing. The problem occurs when the system does not work normally and those with infections have a greater difficulty in controlling them. This process is seen in chronic granulomatous disease and in people with inherited defects in producing some of the complement components. These individuals will thus have greater risk of certain types of infections.[1]

In the acute inflammatory process, the pathogens are either bacteria, viruses, or some dramatically injured tissues. The major cells involved are primarily neutrophils and some basophils. Eosinophils would be present if there were parasites or worms that were causing the infection. The primary mediators of the acute inflammatory process are monocytes and macrophages. The mediators (compounds) they produce are primarily vasoactive amines and eicosanoids. These create blood vessel dilation and leaking into the tissues. In this type of inflammation, the onset is immediate, and the typical duration will be a few days, leading to abscess formation. If not resolved, chronic inflammation is the result.

During the acute phase of inflammation, marked vascular changes occur where the vessels become more open, resulting in increased permeability through the walls and an increase in blood flow. The inflammatory mediator cytokines and other products previously discussed create these changes. The vasodilation begins in the capillary beds, increasing to larger and larger vessels, which helps to create the redness, heat, and swelling of inflammation. This increased permeability allows plasma to move into the other tissues with resultant stasis. As the blood vessels dilate, cells move from the center of the blood vessel to the periphery, along the walls. The endothelial cells of the vessel walls are coated with chemoattractants on their surface, and these cause the blood cells to move to the edges, slowing movement, and then to traverse the vessel cell wall between the endothelial cells.[1,4,20,22]

These activities attract and direct cells into the inflamed tissues. The leukocytes in the bloodstream begin to slow and move to the margins of the blood vessels. As this occurs, they begin to roll slowly and then penetrate between the endothelial cells and move into the tissues. Known as the leukocyte adhesion cascade,[23] cells migrate into the tissue and the whole process of inflammation is carried out.

The resolution of inflammation is an active process. Inflammation needs to be ended when the inciting cause has been taken care of and there is no other tissue at the present time. When this process is working correctly, neighboring tissue is not damaged and the inflammation is resolved. If this process does not end correctly, chronic inflammation and cellular destruction ensues.[22] The different mechanisms for resolving inflammation will be determined by the type of tissue where the inflammation is taking place.[22,24] One of the contributing factors to the resolution of inflammation is that the inflammatory mediators are decreased in the tissue. This is followed by a reduction in the macrophage activation and production and release of transforming growth factor-beta (TGF-beta), which comes from the macrophage itself.[25,27] TGF-beta is produced with a reduction in the TNF-alpha production and a shift to TGF-beta.

If this process doesn't occur, and the macrophages continue to produce TNF-alpha, the inflammatory process will continue and expand. At other times, the production and release of interleukin-10 (IL-10)[28] functions to reduce inflammation. The production of anti-inflammatory lipoxins[29] can act as down regulators of the proinflammatory molecules such as leukotrenes. In addition, an up-regulation of anti-inflammatory molecules, such as Interleukin-1 receptor antagonists, or production of soluble tumor necrosis factor receptors can lead to the apoptosis of proinflammatory cells,[30] leading to the end of the inflammatory reaction.

If an inflammatory reaction progresses for an extended period of time, some receptors are desensitized. An increase in inflammatory cells in the inflamed area will lead to a continued interaction with the extracellular matrix (ECM);[31,32] with the increase in cells and ligands, the receptors reach a point of saturation and they then begin to down-regulate. There can also be cleavage of some chemokines by the matrix metallopreotieases (MMPs) and the subsequent production of anti-inflammatory factors.[33]

In the case of chronic inflammation, the inflammatory process rages out of proportion to the threat, or it may be directed against inappropriate targets. This can lead to more damage to the body and be even greater than the threat from the triggering agent itself. All allergies and many autoimmune diseases are examples of this type of reaction. The formation of antibodies against "self" or persistent antigens from a smoldering infection can, in some cases, make the problem worse. In these cases, a formation of antibody complexes act to trigger the complement system and create more mediators of inflammation.[1]

Persistent acute inflammation, nondegradable pathogens, viral infections, persistent foreign bodies, or an autoimmune reaction can result in chronic inflammation. The cells involved tend to be mononuclear cells, such as monocytes, macrophages, lymphocytes, plasma cells and fibroblasts. In chronic inflammation, some of the primary mediators are interferon gamma (IFN-gamma), cytokines, growth factors, ROS, and hydrolytic enzymes. This whole process is delayed and may last up to months or years, creating tissue destruction fibrosis and necrosis.[22]

As one begins to understand the complexity of the process and resolution of inflammation, it becomes increasingly clear that there must be things we can to prevent this process from even starting and continuing. At the core of everything we do to maintain our health is diet. We can eat things that are pro-inflammatory, or we can eat things that help reduce inflammation. We can take supplements, for example, that will help to prevent and control chronic inflammation. The current American diet is filled with processed food and genetically modified food and is, overall, very acidic. Processed oils tend to increase the process of inflammation, as well as fatty meats and dairy, foods with trans-fats, sugars and other sweeteners, and flour containing genetically modified gluten. The simple-carbohydrate foods also contribute to inflammation, including white rice, as do omega-6 oils, some peppers, tomatoes, and eggplant. These can all contribute to increase and propel inflammation.[34]

Rather than avoiding all of these foods, we need to choose foods that are alkaline and provide our body with what it needs to control inflammation. Spices such as turmeric or curcumin help to control inflammation. Complex carbohydrates, such as fruits and vegetables, are more beneficial for our body than simple carbohydrates. Lacto-fermented foods, such as pickles and beet kvass, provide us with probiotics, digestive enzymes, vitamins, and minerals. These foods, along with natural supplements, help us to control inflammation.

As we look at diet in our lives, we can draw one conclusion: The commonality between all of our chronic diseases is inflammation, and inflammation itself is a link to our diet. Our diet, therefore, is one of the first things that we need to change.

The plant *Cannabis sativa*, as described in chapter 1, is one of the oldest and most studied of the natural substances. It provides phytocannabinoids, some of which contain antioxidants, are anti-inflammatory and neuroprotective, and can help us to control chronic inflammation. Cannabidiol (CBD) is one of the phytocannabinoids, an antioxidant that acts as an immune modulator, is anti-inflammatory and protects mitochondria from damage. Nonpsychoactive, CBD is used to help control seizures and antitumor activity and can turn off genes for the metastasis of some tumors.

In this book we look at many of CBD's applications and the methods by which anyone can accomplish these goals for health. *Cannabis sativa* is a natural herb. It grows on this earth for our benefit. Hopefully, we as a society will begin to look at it again, to understand how to use it for our benefit. It has the potential to benefit anyone who has chronic inflammation. CBD can aid and assist in reducing inflammation and protecting the cells that surround the area of inflammation in any system, organ, or tissue. Since most diseases are associated with chronic inflammation, using CBD enables us to intervene to reduce the inflammation and protect the neighboring undamaged cells.

III

The Endocannabinoid System

The endocannabinoid system is designed to maintain homeostasis balance in our bodies.[1] It interconnects all systems, organs, and tissues and responds to changes in the internal and external environment. Its whole purpose is to keep our bodies functioning at their best by adapting to change. When the endocannabinoid system is working correctly, we are in balance and function at our maximum potential. When this system is underresponding or overresponding, we begin to have physical and mental issues.

The endocannabinoid system is based on lipid mediators[73] that are metabolized on an as-needed basis. The compounds are quickly made and broken down. Their function is to help us respond to stress by modulating the endocrine system's response to environmental changes. They also help us to modulate inflammation in the body and to regulate our fight-or-flight response.

The trigger for learning about cannabinoids came from the experiences with phytocannabinoids, cannabinoids that are derived from plants. Of particular interest was the action of delta-9-THC from the marijuana plant. As they speculated on how THC produced its psychotropic effects, chemists began to look at the plant and discovered more than 60 cannabinoids. Research continues on the effects of each of these phytocannabinoids on our body.

In 1963 the structure of CBD was discovered,[2] followed in 1964 with the discovery of the structure of the psycho-active compound in marijuana. It was first called delta-1-tetrahydrocannabinol and the nomenclature was later changed to delta-9-THC.[3] From this research it became evident that our cells had some way to interact and respond to the cannabinoids. In 1988 a cannabinoid receptor was discovered in the rat brain.[4] The receptors were part of the Gi/o family of G-protein coupled receptors and similar to many other receptors in our body. These receptors help modulate ion channels, the calcium and potassium channels that move these ions in and out of cells. These channels help modulate neurotransmission.[12] Many hormones act through G-protein coupled receptors.[11]

In 1990 the cannabinoid receptor type 1 (CB1) was cloned.[5] This receptor was found expressed in the central nervous system (CNS) and other tissues and organs in the body. There are a few CB1 receptors in the medulla oblongata, so they do not regulate respiration and cardiovascular function. This precludes a reaction of respiratory failure or cardiovascular collapse from marijuana consumption.[11] The receptors were also found in the cardiovascular system, the reproductive system in both males and females,[11] and the gastrointestinal tract.[13] It was discovered that this CB1 receptor is responsible for the psycho-trophic activity of delta-9-THC.

A high density of CB1 receptors exists in the basal ganglia, especially the globus pallidus, which helps control unconscious muscle movements, and planning and starting a movement.[14-16] A high concentration also exists in the limbic system. In the amygdala, these receptors influence emotion, such as fear and anxiety, and this is paired with a high number of CB1 receptors in the hippocampus, which is involved in learning new information and memory integration.[14-16] In the cerebellum, these receptors affect motor coordination and balance. In the brain stem they affect the transmission of information from the brain to the spinal column and the spinal column to the brain. This area also helps control nausea. The cannabinoid receptors in the hypothalamus help modulate eating and sexual behavior. Those in the neocortex and forebrain support complex thinking and higher cognitive function, feeling, and movement.[15] The cannabinoid receptors in the nucleus accumbens modulate motivation and reward. Some of the cannabinoid receptors in the spinal cord regulate the transmission between the body and the brain, modulating pain sensitivity and perception.

The CB1 receptors are located presynaptically, and the endocannabinoids are made in response to the neuron firing. They are made in the postsynaptic membrane and then move in a retrograde manner to affect the firing of the presynaptic membrane. They will help modulate what neurotransmitter is released and how quickly the neuron can fire.[31,39,40] The CB1 receptors are associated with special microdomains called lipid rafts. These lipid rafts respond to changes in cholesterol levels. With increased cholesterol levels, they reduce binding to the CB1 receptors. They also help modulate endocannabinoid signaling.[86-88]

In 1992 the first endocannabinoid was discovered[6] and named anandamide, meaning "internal bliss." The chemical name was N-arachidonoyl ethanolamide (AEA). The next step in discovery was identifying receptors for cannabinoids and the presence of the first endocannabinoid. Anandamide is a modified form of arachidonic acid, a compound synthesized by the enzyme N-acylphosphatidylethanolamine-specific phospholipase D (NAPE-PLD).[75-76] The structure of this compound is different from THC and functions in both the central and peripheral nervous systems. There is a cross-tolerance to THC;[19] both THC and anandamide increase the affinity and number of cerebellar and hippocampal receptors after acute and chronic use.[20] Both of these compounds are strong CB1 receptor agonists and weak CB2 receptor agonists. After its use, the anandamide is degraded by fatty acid amide hydrolase (FAAH), breaking it down to arachidonic acid and ethanolamide. FAAH is the enzyme that degrades some of our endocannabinoids. Anandamide acting at CB1 receptors provides neuromodulatory function. Unlike other neuromodulatory molecules, it is produced in the postsynaptic membranes in response to its firing. Nerve impulses move from the presynaptic membrane across the synaptic cleft to stimulate the post-synaptic membrane. When this occurs, anandamide is produced and moves in the reverse direction from the post-synaptic membrane to the CB receptor on the presynaptic membrane. This interaction modulates the Ca2+ and K+ ion movement and stimulates adenylyl cyclase activity. Through this activity, it modulates the neurotransmitter release.[84]

The discovery of anandamide was followed in 1993 with the cloning of a second type of cannabinoid receptor, endocannabinoid receptor 2 (CB2).[7] This receptor was found in peripheral tissues and organs, principally in immune system cells, and a second isoform was later found to be present and active in the CNS central nervous system.[10] The CB2A isoform has higher concentration in the testis and the brain, while the CB2B has a higher expression in the peripheral tissues.[10h]

The CB2 receptors were found in the cerebral cortex in the orbital, visual, motor, and auditory areas. They were also found in the hippocampus, both CA2 and CA3 areas, the corpus collosum, cerebellum, brain stem, and pineal gland.[10] Peripherally they were found in the marginal zone of the spleen,[11] in the immune system, in the lymphocytes, macrophages, NK cells, and other immunocytes.[17] From this distribution the CB2 receptors can modify brain function and immune function. CB2 receptors were also found in the enteric nervous system, which helps modulate gastrointestinal contractility.[18]

In 1995 a second endocannabinoid was discovered and named 2-arachidonoyl glycerol (2-AG). 2-AG is more CB2 receptor-selective, as it will bind to both CB1 and CB2 receptors.[8,9] It is produced more in peripheral tissues and was first discovered in canine tissues.[21] It is also derived from arachidonic acid and is synthesized by a phospholipase C compound—sn-1-diacylglycerol lipase (DAGL)[77] and is broken down by monoacylglycerol lipase (MAGL).[78] It has a similar activity to THC in peripheral tissues. Several other endocannabinoids have been described, including palmitoyl-ethanolamide (PEA), docosatetraenylethanolamide (DEA), homo-gamma-linoenylethanolamide (HEA), virodhamine, noland ether, oleamide, and oleoylethanolamine (OEA).[73] All of these compounds are a family originating from arachidonic acid and are unsaturated fatty acid ethanolamides that bind to cannabinoid receptors. They can all produce behavioral effects, pain perception modification, learning, memory, and sleep. The activities of the endocannabinoids and phytocannabinoids are not limited to only cannabinoid receptors.

With the discovery of the receptors, it became obvious that we had an endogenous system with receptors and active compounds. The distribution of the receptors indicated that these compounds helped with the modulation of neuropeptides and hormones, and that, through these interactions, the endocannabinoid system helped modulate the regulation of the brain and behavior.[93,96] All of this information came from the study of the herb marijuana and, with it, the discovery of a complete system that functions to help us stay in balance. The endocannabinoid system affects all systems, organs, and tissues, so when it is out of balance, we are out of balance and disease develops. The illnesses can be from too little or too much cannabinoid tone (the baseline amounts of endocannabinoids produced. Most people have not had their cannabinoid system supplemented since they were breast-fed. If they were not breast-fed, this system has not been supported since birth.

IV

Anxiety

Anxiety is the most common diagnosis given today, so prevalent that its treatment now supports multiple medications. Anxiety is a complicated physiological process, and, through experimentation, we have learned much about which parts of the brain are active in anxiety. Anxiety is different for each person experiencing it. It can be perceptual in that some things that produce anxiety for one person may not create it for someone else. Anxiety is dependent on a person's interpretation of another person, place, or event. Something that seems perfectly normal to one person might appear to be threatening and overwhelming to another. Complicating factors for anxiety are those instances that might not be an event that is actually happening but rather anticipation or worry about possible events or even an inward interpretation of an event that is happening. These are reflections of our individuality, and their complexity is important to understand.

Anxiety has specific triggers, and, as these triggers are processed, they can be generalized and create even more triggers. This can happen with thoughts that create anxiety, and the thoughts then become obsessive and repetitive. I believe the obsessive complex begins to develop to help reduce anxiety. For many children on the autistic spectrum, for example, the obsessive-compulsive activities start from a core of anxiety or fear.

Recurrent thoughts or repetitive activities help some people reduce the level of anxiety or fear. They provide a method of coping with the anxiety or fear by giving them something they can control. This brings to mind the whole flight-or-fight mechanism. When fearful or anxious emotions are present, our body is in a constant state of readiness to either fight or run. Cortisol levels are elevated, the heart rate increases, breathing is rapid and shallow, and the body becomes dependent on the subsequent adrenaline rush. If this dependency is developed, then there is gravitation toward similar situations that create the same feeling. Situations are modified to become fulfilling.

The whole cycle may become self-reinforcing and repetitive, and from this long-term place of constant elevated stress reaction, the body's overall function is unbalanced. Anxiety shuts down the frontal cortex, leading to reduced memory and reduced executive functions. It's not difficult to understand that anxiety makes it difficult to cope and successfully thrive in our society. In everyday life, we need to be remembering and processing nearly constantly, and none of these functions are maximal when we are experiencing anxiety. The greater the anxiety, the less we are able to function, and our ability to function from moment to moment is decreased. By just living life, we are then creating more and more triggers for more anxiety. When this occurs in early life, education is severely affected, not just in the classroom but in social education as well. When widespread, this anxiety can make even leaving the house intolerable.

Triggers for anxiety are personal, so understanding their origin or starting place is difficult. Since the triggers in the whole process are individualized, we must approach each person differently and use personalized therapeutic interventions. When developing a treatment plan, one must understand the areas of the brain involved and the balance of the neurotransmitters. One must begin with underlying support of the natural processes that help reduce anxiety.

Our microbiota has a tremendous influence on how we react to stress and therefore influence anxiety. This appears to be a starting place as microbiota accounts for 80 percent of our innate immune system. Our microbiota helps produce our neurotransmitters, serotonin, and dopamine. Our microbiota also helps influence our hypothalamic pituitary adrenal (HPA) axis in its response to stress. The connection between our gut and brain is a powerful one, and microbiology even influences calm and aggressive behaviors. We must approach anxiety from the basis of the microbiota and its influence on the body.

Our body works as a whole and not in isolated segments or sections. Understanding this and understanding multiple interactions enables us to further hone the approach to working with anxiety. To calm the anxiety, we basically must start from the ground and work our way up. We cannot expect to just treat symptoms and have anxiety go away. The approach must include looking for those pieces that are out of balance, moving from the basic to the more complex. This is where CBD can be of great value.

CBD helps to calm anxiety by working in different parts of the brain where the anxiety starts and helping one to release triggers. This is accomplished with low doses; when doses get too high, anxiety may increase. When treating anxiety with CBD, we start with the basics and move up. When started at low doses and gradually worked up, CBD has no psychotropic effects. If large doses are given at the start, CBD can block the reuptake and degradation of our own CB1 receptor agonist, anandamide, and cause a feeling of spaciness. Nonetheless, the safety profile of CBD is extraordinary, and, with proper use, it can be very effective in treating anxiety in young people without creating any problems. Since there are no cannabinoid receptors in the respiratory and cardiovascular nuclei in the brain stem, death is not a risk in taking cannabinoids. The biggest side effects are "the munchies" and sleepiness.

The limbic system functions in disorders related to anxiety and stress,[1] helping to mediate emotional learning[2,8-15] and affecting and interacting with the complete neurophysiological system of stress, anxiety, and fear.[1] The endocannabinoid system helps us to modulate our stress reactions and is heavily expressed in brain areas associated with stress, fear, emotion, and reward, such as the amygdala, the nucleus accumbens (NAc), the hippocampus, and the prefrontal cortex (PFC).[3-7]

Stress is defined as any situation that challenges the homeostasis of the organism and may be perceived as actual or potential changes in the individual's environment. These may be real or perceived,[18] and a dynamic endocannabinoid system helps regulate or modulate the HPA axis system. The endocannabinoid system thus helps regulate a stress response, anxiety, and the extinction of fear learning.[8, 19, 20] Fear is an adaptive component of the acute stress response or reaction when we are faced with potentially dangerous situations or environments.[1] When fear is disproportionate in intensity or chronicity, is irreversible, or is not associated with any actual risk, then it is considered maladaptive and can lead to anxiety-related psychiatric disorders.[20] The brain regions involved in stress, anxiety, and posttraumatic stress disorder (PTSD) include the amygdala, the prefrontal cortex, and the hippocampus.[21]

The hippocampus contains large numbers of both mineralocorticoid and glucocorticoid receptors.[22] Stress-induced corticosteroids signaling in the hippocampus have a beneficial role in regulating the time course of the HPA axis stress response,[22] but prolonged glucocorticoid signaling can damage the hippocampus, causing dendritic atrophy, decreased neurogenesis, and deficits in synaptic plasticity.[23-26] In PTSD and major depressive disorder, patients' hippocampal volumes are reduced,[27-29] and smaller hippocampal volumes are predictive of vulnerability to the development of stress-related disorders and depression.[30]

The amygdala has a central role in the control of emotions and autonomic responses to stress, mood regulation, and mediation of fear and stress responses.[31,32] There is a bidirectional relationship with the frontal cortex[33] and hippocampus.[34] Each has influence on the other, both in forming and releasing stress responses. The human amygdala is responsive to a multitude of salient stimuli, such as fear conditioning, emotional stimuli, and facial expressions. However, it responds reliably and potentially preferably to stimuli that project threat and can be involved in mediating fear and anxiety states.

The experience of fear as a "distress response" to possible predictors of threat is present in anxiety disorders. The amygdala is hypothesized to be hyperresponsive in some stress reactions. A reaction follows that may create hyperresponsive reaction in some anxiety disorders. Scientists have proposed that the amygdala is hyperresponsive in PTSD and that it's this hyperresponsiveness that accounts for the exaggerated response to, and persistence of, traumatic memories.[21]

The prefrontal cortex has an integral role in mediating a range of executive functions that subserve the selection and processing of information necessary to plan, control, and direct behavior in a manner appropriate to the current environmental demands.[35-40] This is an area where an imbalance in the endocannabinoid system will show in many inappropriate or disproportionate reactions to some situations. The prefrontal cortex plays a major role in orchestrating behavioral and systemic responses to stress. Neurons of the prefrontal cortex in rats have extensive remodeling in response to stress. Stress-induced alterations in the prefrontal cortex function represent the principal neural insult from stress and lead to deficits in executive function in rodents and to many neuropsychiatric diseases[41] in humans. In addition, the amygdala and hippocampus establish roles in encoding and processing memory for emotional stressful events into long-term storage.[42-49]

The NAc is involved in mediating stress-related dysfunction.[50-52] The shell of the NAc has an important role in integrating and consolidating representations of new experiences that are initially processed by both the amygdala and hippocampus.[53-55] The shell of the NAc receives neural input from the basal lateral amygdala concerning the effective components of the experiences[56,57] and is the "emotional" content of the new experiences.

Projections from the hippocampus, ventral subiculum region, convey information about the context of events occurring in the environment, along with reward-related components of learning experiences from the ventral tegmental area. Contextual features would look at permanence, transient features, relevance to the whole situation, and whether this has a possibility of recurrence.[60] The interconnecting of multiple areas allows the endocannabinoid system to modulate unconditioned stress- and anxiety-like responses.[8,11,13] Inhibition of the interconnecting signaling increases stress and anxiety, and moderate increases in the signaling decreases stress and anxiety.[13] High increases in CB1 receptor stimulation will increase stress and anxiety-like responses.[13,61,62] Endocannabinoids have a biphasic response; low doses are anxiolytic and high doses can be anxiogenic.[14,63] Low doses reduce anxiety and stress, while moderate to high doses increase anxiety and stress responses.

Cannabis may induce aversive states in some people, and even anxiety or panic attacks.[64] The administration of THC may result in psychotic-like states.[65] With the biphasic effect, low doses of CB1 receptor agonist are helping to release the triggers, while high doses can increase aversion and anxiety-related behaviors.[8]

At higher doses, the CB1 receptor agonists begin to stimulate transient receptor potential vallanoid type 1 (TRPV1).[66] This may participate in the negative effects of higher doses. CBD also stimulates TRPV2 receptors, located on afferent nocioceptors. This means that they participate in the transduction of chemical, thermal, and mechanical stimuli. The TRPV1 receptors are located in the hypothalamus, cerebellum, hippocampus and frontal cortex, and play a significant role in inflammation and neurodegeneration.[100] They also play a role in the modulation of the limbic emotional response to fear and anxiety. TRPV2 receptors contribute to ionized calcium (Ca^{2+}) influx, modulate sensitivity for cytotoxic compounds, and help to regulate apoptosis.[98-100]

Anandamide is our normal and natural CB1 receptor agonist; an increased concentration of anandamide will affect not only the CB1 receptors but also begin to affect the TRPV1 receptors. Part of the action of CBD is to block the reuptake and breakdown of anandamide. This is part of the reason that CBD has a biphasic response, reducing anxiety at low levels and increasing anxiety at high levels. Due to the increase in anandamide and its effect on CB1 receptors, CBD can assist in PTSD therapy by helping to release the triggering memories.

The action of CBD is partially related to its ability to reduce the enzyme FAAH, and it further acts by blocking the reuptake protein that removes anandamide from the receptors.[67] Anxiety disorders, including PTSD and phobias, are the result of dysregulation of the neural circuitry controlled by the endocannabinoid system.[68] This imbalance can be improved and reversed by the use of phytocannabinoids and, in particular, CBD.

Using conditioned fear in animals has been a way to understand the mechanism by which aversive memories are formed[1,68] and then understanding the basis for PTSD and specific phobias. By blocking CB1 receptor activity or antagonizing CB1 receptors, we see an increase in the acquisition and expression of "cue" fear conditioning.[69,70] When CB1 receptors are antagonized in the basolateral amygdala, the fear response and conditioning increases, demonstrating that the "cue" fear conditioning depends on the amygdala and not the hippocampus.[12, 71] Blocking or inhibiting the endocannabinoid systems increases fear; moderate stimulation will decrease fear.[1]

An inability to extinguish memories of fear is at the root of all fear disorders, including panic attacks, phobias, and PTSD.[72-74] Extinction learning involves the ventromedial prefrontal cortex, amygdala, and hippocampus.[47,75,76] The lack of CB1 receptor stimuli allows acquisition and consolidation of fear conditioning and also impairs fear extinction.[2,63,77-81] Given this complexity, an individual may need more or less CB1 receptor activity, requiring a combination of CBD and THC in different percentages or ratios.

The activation of the cannabinoid CB1 receptor promotes extinction of our fear memories.[75] The inhibition of FAAH enhances the rate of extinction[82] by increasing the amount of anandamide and activity at CB1 receptors, which is accomplished with CBD. Anxiety responses and fear learning are affected by the endocannabinoid system. This system acts on the amygdala in the lateral basal nuclei, which has high concentrations of CB1 receptors.[83] For these reasons, CBD activity is complicated. It is a weak CB1 receptor antagonist, but at the same time it blocks the activity of FAHH and thereby increases anandamide, which is a CB1 receptor agonist. These pieces point to the need for knowing or appreciating the individuality of the possible responses.

Extinction of averse memories depends on cannabinoid receptors and signaling within the basal lateral amygdala, which then goes to the prefrontal cortex.[2,9,84] The activation of CB1 receptors decreases anxiety responses and amygdala activation to averse stimuli by modulating the cannabinoid firing in the basal lateral amygdala.[85,86]Acute stress enhances the condition avoidance and impairs inhibitory avoidance extension.[12] This reflects a balance that must be maintained, because too much stimulation on either side can create issues with anxiety and fear. With the cannabinoid stimulation, we can prevent stress-induced conditioned avoidance and reduce the retention of the important trigger event. CB1 activity in basal lateral amygdala also contributes to alterations in the HPA axis.[12]

The HPA activation, through CB1 receptors, reduces the production and release of corticosteroid production and modulates both basal HPA axis activity and fine tuning of a stress response.[87] HPA axis response to stress is the acute release of corticotropin releasing factor (CRF), released into the portal system by neurons in the periventricular nucleus (PVN). The corticotropin releasing factor induces the release of adrenocorticotropic hormone (ACTH) from the pituitary. ACTH stimulates the production of glucocorticoids (corticosterone in rats or cortisol in humans) in the adrenal gland. The glucocorticoids have a wide range of effects on the cardiovascular system, the immune system, the metabolic system, and the neural systems, which in turn induces the optimal response to a personal stimulus, as multiple people can be in the same environment and each have their own personal experience or interpretation of the events which occurred.[88] This is the basis of the fight-or-flight response. In an acute situation, this can be protective; however, on a long-term basis, this is destructive, causing more problems than it solves.

Cortisone also exerts negative feedback for the HPA axis, inhibiting the further release of CRF and ACTH from the axis. The amygdala activates the HPA axis,[1, 88] while the hippocampus and prefrontal cortex inhibit it[1,88] Stressful events cause an increase in the endocannabinoid stimulation in several brain areas in response to the stimulation of glucocorticoid receptors.[89,90] Stress stimulates and increases endocannabinoid production in the periaqueductal gray matter in the midbrain.[91] Stress causes changes in the endocannabinoid system in the limbic forebrain, the amygdala, stratum, and in the prefrontal cortex.[86,92]

CBD blocks transporter protein for anandamide, blocks FAAH breakdown of anandamide, or both, which in turn reduces corticosteroid release in stress-induced reactions[93.] This increase in anandamide is accompanied by the administration of CBD. This also reduces activation of the HPA axis and the cannabinoids' negative modulation of the axis. Stress itself induces a reduction in the endogenous anandamide present in the amygdala through an increase in FAAH activity.[86,92,94] This is one of the places where CBD can help to control the stress response.

CB1 receptor agonists have a biphasic activity with regard to anxiety-like behaviors in the HPA axis activation. Low doses reduce anxiety and reduce corticosteroid release. The endocannabinoid system is an important regulator of the central stress response, and alterations of the cannabinoids help reduce stress responses and prevent stress-related diseases.

CB1 receptor agonists also reduce gamma-aminobutyric acid (GABA) in the basal lateral amygdala interneurons, reducing inhibition of the GABAergic neurons in the intercolated nuclei. This increases their inhibition of the parental neurons in the central amygdala.[83] Reduction in this inhibitory tone may indirectly reduce anxiety by increasing the activity of the hippocampus and forebrain and inhibit the activation of the central amygdala.[83]

Cannabinoids decrease CRH levels in the central amygdala, which is associated with decreases in aversive stress responses.[61] There may also be interactions with other neurochemicals, such as serotonin, cholecystokinin, and opioids.[95] Moderate stress, learning, extension of the fear, and emotional learning reward processes are associated with functions of the amygdala and hippocampus NAc and the prefrontal cortex.[96] Stimulation of these areas causes a reduction in anxiety and some antidepressant activity.[66,97-99] CB1 receptors are required for neuronal emotional learning and memory,[9] and are essential for the extinction of conditioned fear.[100] The blocking of CB1 receptors completely blocks emotional learning.

CBD's action is not through the cannabinoids receptors. CBD is a reverse agonist of CB1 receptors and is a weak agonist. Part of its effectiveness against anxiety is through its ability to block FAAH in the protein reuptake for anandamide. Anandamide is our natural CB1 receptor agonist. Through modulation, we get either increase or decrease anxiety. With the biphasic activity, we must remember that, at higher doses, we will increase anxiety rather than reduce it.

This activity is mainly seen in the amygdala, hippocampus, and prefrontal cortex. CBD has benefits other than just calming anxiety. The help with releasing triggers has been shown to have some benefit with PTSD. Through modulation, CBD is a very effective anxioloytic with no psychotropic effects. With the proper therapy and use of low doses of CBD, traumatic memories are released and normal function can return. Understanding that CBD is just one of many cannabinoids, we can surmise that research will show that combinations of cannabinoids will give us greater benefits than any one by itself.

Many additional valuable and holistic approaches and therapies can be used to calm anxiety. One of the best resources for these is a book called *Freedom from Anxiety* by Marcie Shapiro.

V

Immune System

Our immune system is complex and serves us in many capacities. It protects us from invasion from the outside by microorganisms and, on the inside, by clearing out damaged cells. It is balanced between two sides, the Th1 and the Th2. The activity it carries out shifts between them, with the Th1 as the clearing, antiviral and anticancer side, and the Th2 the antibody-producing side.

This system has to be in balance and able to shift back and forth, like a teeter-totter: when one side is active, the other side is suppressed. If the system becomes locked into one side, the other side does not function. The shifts can be caused by recurrent infections, heavy metals, or genetic predispositions. A look into the diseases reveals that chronic inflammation is at the base of the problem.

Chronic inflammation sets up a chronic shift in the immune system. This shift is on the Th1 side, where the promotion of cytokines produced at the site of inflammation are preventing the immune response from shifting. When this occurs in a particular area, the cells become damaged, more immune cells are called into the area. The immune cells become activated and start producing more inflammatory cytokines, which continue the immune response. If the response continues to escalate, the damaged cells are not removed or repaired but the damage begins to spread and affect the surrounding cells.

The triggers for this process are varied and multiple. Looking at the diseases reviewed in this chapter, we can see that each type has its own specific trigger or cause. In the big picture, it comes down to the question of whether someone suffering from one of these diseases can help remediate the problem and modulate the immune system. To help modulate the immune system, the patient has to be able to turn off the inflammatory promoting cytokines. The cytokines are the controllers of immune system function. These compounds travel through the blood stream and function throughout the whole body. When inflammation is established in one area, the whole body knows and begins to respond.

Interferon and multiple cytokines, chemokines, and interleukins have specific functions. Some recruit more immune cells, some provide a trail for immune cells to follow, and some activate new recruited immune cells. Each immune cell has its own function and when a cell becomes activated, it will begin to provide its particular abilities to the area where it has been summoned. Some will attack, ingest, and destroy a bacteria or a virus. Others will present the markers of the invader and then present these to other immune cells that can produce antibodies. Still other immune-system cells will attack and destroy cells that have viruses or microbes in them. These cells will also attack cancer cells.

In autoimmune and neuroinflammatory disease, there is a Th1 shift. This shift is maintained and escalated by repeated and persistent presence of Th1 cytokines, chemokines, and interleukins. As long as these are present, the process is reinforcing and expanding. It must be broken by a modification in cell activation and reduction, or a change in the cytokine and interleukin profile. The common stimulators of this Th1 side include interferon-gamma, interleukin-2 (IL-2), TNF-alpha, and lymphotoxin. When these are continually made, the inflammatory process will continue and inflammation will spread and result in tissue damage from cell destruction.

This is the process that is seen in autoimmune and neuroinflammatory diseases. Control over these cytokines and interleukins can mean the progression or the cessation of the disease. When one looks at the activity of phytocannabinoids, it is obvious that they can be helpful in controlling the Th1 shift and begin to give support to end the Th1 cycle of destruction. CBD has been shown to reduce the production and release of TNF-alpha from arthritic synovial cells.[2] Part of the decrease in the production of TNF-alpha came from the stimulation of adenosine A2A receptors.[3] CBD has also been shown to reduce the production of interleukin-8 (IL-8) and other chemokines, thereby suppressing human B cell activities.[2,62,63]

CBD has also been shown to reduce the release of ROS, demonstrated in zymosin-stimulating neutrophils.[2] It was also demonstrated that CBD can reduce nitric oxide production in macrophages.[2] All of these activities are helping to reduce oxidative stress and immune imbalance. The cannabinoids have also been shown to reduce the production of interleukin 10 (IL-10) through the cannabinoid receptors, seen in both macrophages and splenocytes.[2] The capabilities of cannabinoids can help reduce all of the proinflammatory cytokines, interleukins, chemokines, and interferon that support a Th1 shift.[2-8]

A wide distribution of CB2 receptors exists in immune cells.[10-15] CBD has been shown to block the production of antigen-specific antibodies and can suppress T cell proliferation and the production of interleukin-2, interleukin-4 and interferon-gamma.[2,5-7] CBD can also induce cell death in immature immortalized T-cells, an activity produced by the generation of ROS within these cells. CBD has been shown to be effective in the modulation of immune reactions within the central nervous system (CNS). The CB2 receptors are increased in microglial cells when inflammation is present, therefore providing a good opportunity to reduce inflammatory reactions and activation.

It has been shown that the CB2 receptors play a role in B-cell differentiation.[17] These are the cells that produce antibodies. When they are suppressed, the body is more open to some types of infections, including *Legionella pneumophilia*, *Staphylococcus albus*, *Treponema pallidum*, Friend leukemia virus, and *Acanthamoeba* (a protozoa genus).[28,32-36] It has been shown that agonists of the CB2 receptors can suppress the proliferation of both B and T lymphocytes.[37-40] They can also suppress the activity of NK cells,[39] which are the cells that lead to cell destruction and the proliferation of autoimmune diseases or neural inflammation.[39] These compounds have also been shown to reduce the ability of cells to move toward the site of inflammation, therefore reducing immune cell recruitment and limiting injury.[41,42]

The application of exogenous or phytocannabinoids shifts the immune profile from proinflammatory Th1 to two or more antiinflammatory Th2 stances.[17,43-46] Observing the activity that these compounds produce leads to an understanding of the tremendous benefit they provide in helping to control autoimmune disease and neuroinflammation.[47-57] They have the capability of turning off the attack by the immune cells, helping to reduce some of the oxidative stress, and supporting and protecting the normal cells.[58-67]

Understanding the effects of the cannabinoids and cannabinoid agonists leads us to conclude that we have an opportunity for control of diseases for which we have not previously had influence.[68-79] However, we must be cautious and not push the Th2 side of the immune system too far and stimulate the production of more allergic-type diseases.[80-84] As with anything, balance and caution is needed and important. The use of these compounds must be followed by looking at CD lymphocyte subsets and monitoring the Th status of the individual.[85-88]

VI

Seizures

The seizures are complex, with many types and causes. Types include partial seizures, absence seizures, and generalized seizures. Many illnesses—as well as toxic exposures, meningitis, and other infections of the CNS—can cause seizures. Sometimes we know the cause of the seizure, but often we don't. From the perspective of knowing the side effects of current epilepsy medications, and the fact that many seizures are not controlled by them, we look further for other compounds that help us to modulate the seizures. This is where CBD can play an important role. Many patients are helped by CBD alone while others need a combination of CBD and THC. The goal of the physician is to find the exact support that each patient's body needs to help reduce and even stop the seizure activity.

When a patient presents with seizures, doctors need to ask a lot of questions. They need to know when seizures started, how long they last, and what type of seizure the person is experiencing. Seizure activity is influenced by neurotransmitter abnormalities, so understanding these and striving for balance is important. Another issue that can contribute to seizure activity is liver function. If the liver is not working normally and removing toxins, they can build and cause irritation in the brain, leading to seizures. Supporting detoxification is very important. Another basic piece to understanding and treating seizures is supporting and balancing the microbiome. Dysbiosis (an internal microbial imbalance), with the reduction of normal flora and an increase in pathogenic bacteria, can cause or contribute to seizures. We depend on our normal microbiome to help balance the activity and responses of our hypothalamus, pituitary, and adrenal gland. The microbiome also helps to modulate the immune system, another important factor in seizure activity and control. The microbiome provides 80 percent of our innate immune response; the microbes in it are our first responders to the introduction of pathogens. They tell us how the immune system is working, whether there is a Th1 or Th2 shift, or whether the immune system is in neutral and not contributing at all. When the immune system is out of balance, inflammation and seizure activity can be ongoing. Knowing a patient's infectious-disease history is essential to understanding the patient's seizure activity, because bacteria, viruses, and fungi can cause or exacerbate seizure activity, either during or after the infection.

A patient's vaccination history is another important component of understanding seizures. Because of the adjuvants and other compounds in vaccines, vaccines can trigger seizure activity. Heavy metals are toxic to the brain and can affect cellular activity and cause energetic imbalances in the mitochondria. These issues in the mitochondria in turn can contribute to seizure activity. Hydration and mineral status are also very important determinants as these, too, can contribute to seizures. One of the most impressive seizures that I've seen was precipitated by dairy and gluten in the diet. When these proteins are not digested normally, they become neuroactive peptides, which can interfere with neurotransmitter function and interact with opiate receptors and overall brain function.

We are exposed to many toxins in our environment each day and can support our body's detoxification system by helping it to remove toxins. General support needs to be applied first; then we can work toward more specific stratagems as we learn what is going on in the body and instigating seizure activity. Each person reacts uniquely to toxins, and discovering individual triggers is difficult—sometimes impossible.

One of the biggest problems with treating seizures is tailoring treatment to the disease, as the medications prescribed are extremely varied and complex and can cause numerous undesirable side effects. Many of these medications make you drowsy or may decrease your ability to focus and concentrate, which in turn can interfere with schooling and other normal activities. One of the biggest benefits of CBD is that it has no psychotropic effects; therefore, its use in young children can be very helpful. This is especially true for children who cannot understand what you are trying to explain to them about medications, side effects, and psychotropic activity. High doses of THC can and likely will trigger psychotropic activity. This can increase fear, anxiety, or even produce paranoia. This is why I usually start with low-dose CBD on younger children. Whenever possible, the discussion of the medications should be carried out with the child who is receiving them. The goal is to help control seizures without creating other problems for the individual.

One of the biggest contributions CBD can make is through the control of cell excitement. When you can make cells less excitable, you can help to reduce seizure activity. Cannabis has applications for both partial and generalized seizures, and, because CBD is nonpsychotropic, it has low toxicity and a high tolerability in humans.[6] CBD elicits seizure control through multiple mechanisms of modulating neuronal excitability. It exerts a bidirectional regulation of Ca2 plus homeostasis, accomplished through mitochondrial activity that involves Na+/Ca2+ ion exchanges. This activity can either increase or decrease cytosolic calcium levels and will depend on the neurons' activity—either normal physiologic activity or a highly excitable state.[1]

CBD is an agonist or stimulates positive activity at 5-HT1A receptors (HT stands for hydroxytryptamine).[2-6] Activation of these receptors will elicit membrane hyper-polarization, which in turn inhibits seizure generation.[7,8] These receptors are a subset of serotonin receptors.[7,8] CBD further acts by increasing the active adenosine levels in the CNS by reducing the adenosine reuptake.[9,10] The reduction of adenosine reuptake increases the inhibitory adenosinergic tone to help further suppress seizures. CBD also acts as an antagonist at CB1 receptors, inhibiting the presynaptic terminals that may increase GABA release. This in turn helps to decrease endocannabinoid tone and thereby helps increase the level of inhibition for other seizure activity.[11]

Other CBD activity includes the blocking of breakdown of anandamide by FAAH and the reuptake of this compound into the neuron. This activity produces CB1 receptor agonism.[12-14] CBD can also block low-voltage activated (T-type) Ca2+ ion channels, further helping to modulate neuronal excitability.[15] CBD increases and modulates the activity of glycine receptors, which further reduces excitability of the neurons.[16]

In experimental studies, CBD is shown to be effective against grand mal seizures, cortical focus seizures, complex partial seizures, and temporal lobe epilepsy.[6,17] In my practice, I try CBD as a first-line treatment. I have had great success with seizure control with CBD alone. I also have many patients whose seizures have stopped; then slowly, over time, we've been able to reduce and eliminate the seizure medications. What I have seen is that each patient is different, and that we need to work together to eliminate the causes that can be remediated. Looking at the whole individual and addressing any other support needs that they have is imperative.

It is always best to begin with a low dose and then gradually increase. Once you find the sweet spot, the dose will usually be consistent because the body does not build tolerance to CBD. Given the wide variety of seizures, some individuals will require tinctures of both CBD and THC. There are multiple ratios of CBD and THC, and each will have its own efficacy, so we need to work to find the right balance. Fortunately, the CBD helps reduce the psychoactivity of the THC. The higher the amount of THC, the greater the likelihood it will trigger psychoactive reactions, which will limit the efficacy. In many studies, side effects were only seen when THC was used.

I was once asked whether CBD could be used in a particular case of a 17-year-old who had had seizures for 12 years and been on multiple medications. "Frank," as we will refer to him here, had had all the side effects. His history was clean with no big infections, but he did have some anxiety.

My colleagues and I looked at neurotransmitters and they were low. We began to address the neurotransmitter issues and saw a lessening of the anxiety and an improvement in focus and concentration. We then began a low dose of CBD, and the breakthrough seizures Frank was having stopped.

We continued the low dose and then began to reduce one of his medications, slowly tapering it until Frank was no longer getting that medication. He was doing well, with no seizures, and beginning to feel happier and more involved. We began to taper the second medication, and he did well through the first three drops. With the fourth drop, he had a seizure—very short and different from his previous ones.

We then went back up a step on the medication and held there for a couple of weeks. The third week we raised his CBD and waited for two weeks. We then began to taper the medication again. He did well, having no seizures, and the fatigue he'd had for years began to lift. The fatigue was a side effect of the medication. He is now only on CBD and seizure free. He no longer has anxiety, and his focus and concentration are better than ever before.

In sum, each person will respond individually to cannabis, and the dose he or she will need, as well as the particular combinations of CBD and THC, will differ for each individual who has seizures. In addition, medications must be gradually tapered to enable the body to adjust, and no medication should be stopped abruptly.

VII

Neuroprotection

In treating today's neurological diseases need a variety of approaches. Neurological diseases, such as Parkinson's, Huntington's, Alzheimer's, and multiple sclerosis, have some common threads that need to be addressed. Each of these diseases attacks and destroys neurons, creating inflammation in the brain and thus affecting all other systems. One of the major objectives in treating these diseases has to be to protect neurons from damage and to further reduce neuroinflammation. The endocannabinoid system can address several of the prominent issues across these diseases.

The endocannabinoid system is an avenue that supports intercellular communication.[137] The endogenous cannabinoids and phytocannabinoids can provide neural protection.[31,39,114,142] This neural protection is provided through both cannabinoid and noncannabinoid receptors. Their activity with glial cells can provide anti-inflammatory action through the cannabinoid receptors. This activity can help reduce excitotoxicity through the reduction of glutamate release. These compounds also provide mitochondrial stabilization, controlling free cytosol Ca2+ ions. This activity will help both reduce oxidative stress and create better blood supply.

CB2 receptor signaling pathways help reduce cyclic adenosine monophosphate (cAMP)[127] and stimulate prosurvival pathways.

This has been demonstrated in rat oligodendrocytes,[121] in rat RBL2H3M1 mast cells,[131] mouse neural progenators,[120] and the MAPK cascade. Research has shown that CB2 receptor stimulation in rat microglial cells[4] led to cell proliferation and survival of these cells. The same pathway has been demonstrated to help human monocytes[129] and leukemia cells.[130] The same prosurvival pathways have been shown to be activated in many other cell types in the body, including pancreatic cells.[133]

For neuronal protection, CB2 stimulation depends on the cells' differentiation. The reaction to CB2 the reaction to CB2 receptor stimulation will depend on the cells level of differentiation; some cells will go backwards and de-differentiate and move into a proliferative phase, this has been seen in some Glial malignancies and breast cancer.[89,141] In the cancer cells, this stimulation increases death of cancer cells while at the same time protecting normal neuronal cells from damage.

The cannabinoids help modulate the immune system, which is a large contributor to the neuroinflammation and destruction in the neurodegenerative diseases. The cannabinoids can cross the blood-brain barrier and be directed specifically at the CB2 receptors. When there is inflammation in the brain, the number of CB2 receptors on the microglial cells increases; these cells are the generators of the cascade of inflammation.[1] Microglia are macrophage-like cells in the CNS; these cells may participate in the regeneration or the degeneration of the CNS. In the activated state, the cells have specific cell surface receptors; a multitude of different kinds of receptors contribute to their activities, whether inflammatory or anti-inflammatory. When they are activated, they have an increased number of CB2 receptors.

Depending on the stimulation and activation status, these cells can either increase the inflammatory process or they can help to reduce the proinflammatory cytokine production and activation of other cells.[4] The proper stimulation of CB2 receptors can help reduce their proinflammatory activities. There are CB2 receptors on many cell types in the CNS.[11,20,116,120,121] When there is inflammation present, there is an increase in the number of CB2 receptors increases, which can help stop neurodegeneration.[7–12] Diseases in which this would be applicable include multiple sclerosis, amyotrophic lateral sclerosis (ALS), hypoxic-ischemic encephalopathy, Alzheimer's disease, neuropathic pain, and HIV encephalitis.

In this chapter we look at several of these diseases and the activity of cannabinoids. When there is neuroinflammation, there is always an increase in the number of CB2 receptors. However, in early inflammation, there can be a temporary increase in CB1 receptors; in this case, the number is reduced.[15–17] It has been shown that the increase in CB2 receptors occurs early in the process of inflammation.[6, 20–22] This increase in their production has been shown to help reduce the production of proinflammatory cytokines by the microglia.[23–29] So from this research it becomes clear that the CB2 receptors are the ones that can help control the whole neuroinflammatory process.

Some of the neural-protective effects from some of the phytocannabinoids are active through other types of receptors.[31] Some of these compounds can help block the release of glutamate by N-methyl-D-aspartate (NMDA) receptors (NMDARs); by blocking or reducing this release, they decrease the excitement in the neurons and help to reduce neuroinflammation. They can also stimulate the production or release of GABA; this activity may help improve blood supply to the injured brain.[32-34] These cannabinoid compounds also control and help improve glucose utilization, protecting the cells' energy processes.[35, 36] By reducing the amount of glutamate released, these compounds reduce excitotoxicity, thereby helping to save and protect neurons.[32–44] Part of this activity is controlled by CB1 receptors; they act presynaptically to help reduce glutamine release.[43] If the CB1 receptors are blocked, release of glutamate and toxicity can increase;[32, 38, 44] therefore, compounds that stimulate CB1 receptors can increase the neurotoxicity.[45-48]

The cannabinoids help modulate calcium influx, which helps to control glutamate receptors and reduce excitotoxicity.[37] This neural protection is further aided by the antioxidant power of some of the cannabinoids, which reduce oxidative stress.[59, 60] The natural antioxidants that we have—including vitamin A, vitamin C, vitamin E, and ubiquinol—are not present in adequate amounts to handle the increase in free radicals. These ROS are independent of the cannabinoid receptors.[32-34, 60-63] From just its chemistry, CBD is a more potent antioxidant than vitamin C and vitamin E.[63] Therefore, by increasing the endocannabinoid levels and by blocking the reuptake and aggradation, CBD provides excellent antioxidative protection.[64-67]

In all the studies, the phytocannabinoids have been able to reduce inflammation and provide antioxidant protection.[68] In the process of reducing microglia activation, they also reduce the activation and proinflammatory status of astrocytes.[69-76] Astrocytes are deactivated from proinflammatory stimulation and then become quiescent or anti-inflammatory.[70] This is been shown to be supportive in demyelinating diseases, such as multiple sclerosis.[32-77] In all of the neuroinflammatory diseases studied, the cannabinoids have been able to reduce inflammation.[32-34, 49, 69, 78] It has been shown that stimulation of CB2 receptors help reduce neural inflammation and the inflammatory lesions that are produced.[87-93] The lesions are produced from the inflammation destroying neurons.

Many of the cannabinoids have shown the potential to convert an inflammatory process, reducing inflammatory cytokines, and reducing microglial activation, which helps support the survival of astrocytes, oligodendrocytes, and stem cells. This sets the stage for possible repair and regeneration. All of these have been shown to be part of the activity that CBD can accomplish. On each front where neural degeneration occurs, cannabinoids have been shown to reduce damage, protect normal cells, and even protect stem cells and increase regenerative processes. In the following chapters, we look at each of these diseases and explore how these compounds can help reduce the damage that is caused by the disease process itself.

VIII

Alzheimer's Disease

Alzheimer's disease is an age-related neurodegenerative disorder associated with cognitive decline. The disease affects 10 percent of the population over 65 years old and 25 percent of the population over 80 years old.[7] A small proportion of Alzheimer's disease has a genetic basis, while most occurrences are sporadic.[5] The disease is associated with neural inflammation, excitotoxicity and oxidative stress and has several hallmarks.[5, 6, 8]

The first of these hallmarks is the deposition of beta-amyloid proteins called senile plaques. Early in the disease, senile plaques are formed in the hippocampus, cerebral cortex, and amygdala, leading to memory loss and behavioral changes.[10] These plaques are located outside the cells and consist of 1 to 42 amino acid peptides. The abnormal processing of these transmembrane amyloid precursor proteins has the central role in the genesis of Alzheimer's[9] and can evoke neuronal cell death along with the involvement and disruption of cleavage-enzyme activity.[108] Beta-amyloid production acts as a seed for new beta amyloid production.[109]

The immune cells, or microglia, of the brain start to activate and surround the senile plaques, working to clear the beta-amyloid plaque by phagocytosis.[13] They are not capable of completely removing the plaques, though, which leads to their prolonged activation and production of proinflammatory cytokines, such as IL-beta.[14, 15] Local inflammation causes an increase in the processing of amyloid precursor protein, which in the end generates more beta-amyloid.[15]

Activated microglia have direct toxic effects.[16] At the edge of the senile plaque, the cells involved generate ROS that cause oxidative damage to the brain.[13] Damage to cholinergic neurons will affect the brain's activity, and some use of acetylcholinesterase inhibitors will block the breakdown of acetycholine. These compounds only help with mild cognitive impairment.

The second hallmark for the disease is the hyper-phosphory-lation of tau protein producing nitrate tau protein,[6, 106, 107] which may become microtubule-associated proteins.[11]

Chronic inflammation is the third hallmark for Alzheimer's disease. This process leads to activation of both microglial cells and astrocytes. When these cells are activated, they produce and release proinflammatory molecules.[82,83] These molecules perpetuate the reactive gliosis, which can lead to increasing damage and, ultimately, cell death of neighboring neurons. This process leads to expanding and self-perpetuating neuroinflammation.[84] This cycle promotes neuronal death requiring intervention to reduce reactive gliosis and decrease or prevent activation of microglia and astrocytes.

These combined processes evoke activation of the microglial cells, some neuronal cell death, and impaired interneuronal communication. From these two processes, inflammation begins. Nonsteroidal anti-inflammatories in the long term can reduce some risk.[12] They have been shown to slow the onset of disease and may help to reduce the severity. With inflammation, an increase in oxidative stress leads to oxidative damage[116] that can affect lipids, proteins, and nucleic acids. This is also accompanied by a dysregulation of intracellular calcium,[17] excitoxins, and cholinergic neuron damage. These activities also produce mitochondrial defects that lead to the increased production of ROS and reactive nitrogen species (RNS).[110-112] These combined producers of inflammation also lead to an imbalance in transitional metals, including copper, iron, and zinc.[116]

In Alzheimer's disease, there is an up-regulation of microglia in the areas of senile plaques. These cells are producing proinflammatory cytokines and recruiting and activating more immune cells. The microglial cells also have an increased number of CB2 receptors.[26, 28] Activation of cannabinoid receptors and noncannabinoid receptors in the activated glial cells reduces the production of proinflammatory cytokines, which helps reduce the whole inflammatory process.[62] This may be through control or other effects on transcription factors, such as nuclear factor kappa B (NFxB)[56, 63] Cannabinoid receptor stimulation causes a down-regulation of transcription factors involved in the induction of and promotion of inflammation in neurodegenerative diseases. Activation of cannabinoid receptors leads to stimulation in the production of anti-inflammatory cytokines, such as interleukin-1 receptor antagonist (IL-1ra).[64]

Rats with beta-amyloid injections develop inflammation and cognitive impairment. These could be reversed early by using CB1 or CB2 receptor agonists.[26] CB2 receptor stimulation helps to deactivate the activated microglia[26] and increases the removal of beta-amyloid by macrophages.[114] CB2 receptor stimulation can also suppress the immune system.[65]

The endocannabinoid system, with AEA and 2-AG, is in the brain. It contains the enzymes for production, proteins for transport, enzymes for degradation, and CB1 and CB2 receptors. These compounds do not act only on cannabinoid receptors. Dronabiol is an oil-based solution of delta-9-THC,[18] a compound that has been used and shown to decrease disturbed behavior, stimulate appetite, and alleviate nocturnal agitation in some patients.[19]

The cannabinoid system provides antioxidant and anti-inflammatory activity and neuronal protection.[20] CB1 receptors are abundant in the brain, found heavily in the hippocampus, cerebral cortex, and cerebellar basal ganglia.[21] Those found in the hippocampus affect learning and memory[22] and participate in cognitive processes. If they are disrupted early, they will affect neural plasticity. No change has been noted in the number of these receptors near the senile plaque in patients with Alzheimer's.[27, 28]

CB2 receptors are found on neurons in the brain stem[23] and cerebellum[24] and on microglia.[25] In patients with Alzheimer's, an increase in CB2 receptors on the microglia has been noted, as well as in the microglia surrounding a senile plaque.[26] The cannabinoid receptors in the process of Alzheimer's disease become nitrosylated, which impairs their downstream coupling and, therefore, their activity.[26]

FAAH is found to be up-regulated in senile plaques.[28] This enzyme metabolizes anandaminde (AEA), which leads to an increase in anandamide metabolites, such as arachidonic acid. This may also lead to an increase in prostaglandins and other proinflammatory molecules. FAAH in astrocytes leads to the process known as reactive gliosis in the area of beta-amyloid plaques.[29] Neuronal damage increases the production of endocannabinoids.[30, 31] The cannabinoid tone helps influence neuronal survival. Boosting the cannabinoid system can help offer protection against beta-amyloid production and storage.

Beta-amyloid[32] induces hippocampal degeneration and causes gliosis, resulting in cognitive decline. Increased production of 2-AG is the result of cells trying to protect themselves. This increase in production decreases neurotoxicity and prevents memory impairment. Early administration of reuptake inhibitors of anandamide and noland ether, another endocannabinoid, helps reduce beta-amyloid neurotoxicity through the activation of CB1 receptors and the extracellular regulation of kinase pathways.[33]

Memory is affected by events in the hippocampus. Cannabinoids that are CB1 receptor stimulants actually decrease the performance of memory in rodents.[34] This effect is possibly from the reduction in acetylcholine.[35] CB1 receptor antagonists have been shown to improve memory performance.[36] CBD is an antagonist (blocker) of CB1 receptors. Some of the memory impairment that is evoked by beta-amyloid is reversed by cannabinoid antagonism at CB1 receptors.[37] However, the CB1 blockade has been shown to increase the neurodegenerative components.

In Alzheimer's disease there is dysregulation of intracellular Ca2+; this can create excitotoxins within the neurons. There is also excessive activation of NMDARs. These are a subtype of glutamate receptors that when activated, create more excitotoxicity.[38, 39] In the inherited form of Alzheimer's, there is a mutation in the presenilin genes (PS1/PS2) that causes a disruption in calcium signaling.[38] This contributes to neurodegeneration in memory impairment.[40] Beta-amyloid can itself directly increase voltage-dependent Ca2+ channel activity.[41] It can also create Ca2+-permeable pores in the cells.[42] This further increases the intracellular Ca2+ imbalance and is part of the pathologic mechanism.

Beta-amyloid reduces glutamate uptake by astrocytes, which further increases the activation of glutamate receptors and leads to excitotoxicity.[39] Part of the narrow protection that is provided by CBD is from the reduction and control of Ca2+ influx. This process helps reduce or limit the excitotoxicity. Cannabinoids provide some modulation of NMDA receptors[43] and the modulation or inhibition of presynaptic Ca2+ entry.[44, 45] They also suppress excess glutamanergic activity.[46, 47] CB1 receptor activation can inhibit glutamate release and thereby reduce excitotoxicity.[48]

The endocannabinoid production of AEA and 2-AG depend on Ca2+ movement in the postsynaptic cell.[39, 40] The endocannabinoids are produced and provide more feedback control of neurons to reduce excitoxicity.[50] Inhibition of Ca2+ intracellularly is partially controlled by reducing calcium release from ryanodine-sensitive stores.[51] Controlling Ca2+ levels through cannabinoid receptors provides access to a pathway that stimulates production of protein kinase A, reduces production of nitric oxide,[52] and increases brain-derived neurotrophic factor (BDNF). BDNF will increase neurogenesis and help protect neurons against excitotoxicity.[53]

Nonneuronal cells help create the induction of nerve growth factor (NGF). This is induced by cannabinoids acting at CB1 receptors. This stimulation activates several pathways that contribute to neuron protection and CB1 receptor stimulation by 2-AG or anandamide coupling to assist in the production of axonal growth response.[13]

CBD is an antioxidant. It helps to provide neuroprotection against glutamate toxicity.[55] It helps to reduce the induction of inducible nitric oxide synthase (iNOS).[56] It further helps prevent the activation of stress-activated protein kinase p38.[56] It also helps prevent the inflammatory transcription factor, NFxB.[56]

CBD also helps to down-regulate inflammatory signaling with beta-amyloid plaques.[57] This helps reduce beta-amyloid-induced neuronal damage by scavenging ROS and reducing lipid peroxidation. The antioxidant properties are independent of CB1 receptors. CBD can reduce and reverse tau hyperphosphorylation.[58] This is accomplished by reducing phosphorylation of glycogen synthase kinase-3 beta. This is a tau kinase responsible for tau hyperphosphorylation. This works through the Wnt/beta-catenin pathway. Reducing glycogen synthase kinase-3 beta causes a reduction in the amount of precursor protein being converted to form beta-amyloid.[59] This leads to a reduction in the amyloid burden.

CBD can help prevent beta-amyloid effects by reducing tau hyperphosphorylation and oxidative stress, which in turn lead to reducing neuroinflammation and preventing neuronal apoptosis. This compound is devoid of any psychoactivity, and its activities are carried out even when the CB receptors are nitrosylated in the Alzheimer's brain. Since the cannabinoid receptors are not used by CBD, there is no issue with the uncoupling and other downstream activity.[26] The modulation of microglial activity and cell functions do not depend on CB receptors.[115]

CB2 receptors have a large population in microglia,[25] as well as in the neuronal populations in the brain stem and the cerebellum.[24] These receptors influence neuron and other cell survival.[60] Neural protection is assisted through their anti-inflammatory actions.[61] These receptors are up-regulated in activated microglial cells and astrocytes. They help control the local proinflammatory mediator, interleukin-1 beta, as well as ROS and prostaglandins.

Delta-9-THC competitively inhibits acetylcholinesterase.[73,74]This works to increase the amount of acetylcholine and helps reduce beta-amyloid peptide conversion into fibrillar species. It also helps reduce beta-amyloid plaque production. Therefore, cannabinoids can reduce oxidative stress, reduce neural inflammation, and prevent neuronal death. These complications are produced by beta-amyloid. The cannabinoids stimulate the intrinsic healing mechanisms of the brain.

The endocannabinoid system helps regulate neurogenesis.[70-72] Adult neurogenesis is seen in the dentate gyrus of the hippocampus and the subventricular zone.[66] In mouse models of Alzheimer's disease, neurogenesis is reduced,[67] while in postmortem Alzheimer's disease patients there is hippocampal neurogenesis.[68] In animal models, the only things that helped to enhance neurogenesis were dietary restriction and increased BDNF.[69] Both of these led to improved memory.

In addition to helping with neurogenesis regulation, the endocannabinoid system also helps to reduce anxiety and has antidepressant-like effects. These compounds stimulate neuroprogenitor proliferation.[71] They also help with adaptation to neuronal stress by reducing or limiting excitotoxicity. Their potential is in providing long-term progress through neurogenesis.[5]

CBD works in Alzheimer's even though the cannabinoid receptors are modified and not usable. CBD functions through nuclear receptors[77,78] to reduce inflammation, oxidative stress, lipid peroxidation,[57] and neuronal cell death. These nuclear receptors are present in the CNS, and they are increased in Alzheimer's disease.[80,81] CBD further provides stabilization of calcium levels and provides protection for mitochondria. This protection comes through membrane stabilization of the mitochondria, reduction of endoplasmic reticulum stress, and maintenance of cytochrome enzymes so that energy production is continuous and efficient. CBD further helps produce anti-inflammatory effects through adenosine A2A receptors and serotonin 5-HT1A receptors. Through these activities brain function improves.[85-87]

In conclusion, cannabinoids offer some significant help for the Alzheimer's patient. With the present research, there is also an early window for THC to be effective. CBD has been shown to provide support for extended periods of time. It will be interesting to see what new research will provide into the possibilities of the "entourage" effect with other cannabinoids. This research is in its infancy, and the possibilities are endless.

IX

Parkinson's Disease

Parkinson's disease is a form of neural degeneration. The neuropathology exhibits bradykinesia, rigidity, postural instability, and tremor. The tremor and some of the instability are due to the progressive degeneration of dopaminergic neurons in the substantial nigra pars compacta. When these neurons are affected, this leads to a dopaminergic denervation of the stratum.[1,3] Oxidative stress, mitochondrial dysfunction, inflammation, and creation of a metabolic syndrome contribute to the underlying process.[4-6] There is also a further dysfunction of the ubiquitin-Proteasome system[84] and the formation of intracytoplasmic inclusion bodies referred to as Lewy bodies. These are round eosinophilic intracytoplasmic proteinaceious inclusions.[84]

The use of the medication L-dopa as replacement therapy for dopamine loss is the most common treatment used today for mild cases, but over time it induces an irreversible dyskinetic state with involuntary movement.[7] The search at present is for pharmacological interventions that can delay or arrest the progressions of Parkinson's disease.[8,9] The specific goal of these interventions would be to reduce exicitoxicity, modulate calcium influx, reduce oxidative stress, and reduce neuroinflammation.

Cannabinoids provide a method of giving long-term help with protection, and they can also initially enhance motor symptoms.[10-12] Some evidence exists of overactivity of the endocannabinoid transmission in the basal ganglia at some point in Parkinson's disease.[13-15] CBD has been shown to cause an up-regulation of copper-zinc superoxide dismutase. This produces a reduction in oxidative stress and does not depend on the cannabinoid receptor. CBD can provide further neural protection against the progressive degeneration of the nigrostriatal dopaminergic neurons in Parkinson's disease.[16] The mechanisms by which this is accomplished are a combination of several different receptors: cannabinoid, TRPV1, and adenosine A2A.

Neuroprotection in the human basal ganglia has been correlated with the ratio of N-acetylacetate to total creatinine. CBD in the putamen and globis palladus in recreational cannabis users was shown to enhance neuronal and axonal integrity.[18] CBD has been used as an effective antipsychotic in Parkinson's disease at a dose of 150 milligrams (mg) per day and decreased the progression of Parkinson's as well.[19]

CBD provides antioxidant activity from its own chemistry. It provides no protection through peroxisome proliferator-activated receptors (PPARs); these are nuclear receptors that control gene transcription. CBD inhibits caspase 3 generation from its inactive precursor procaspase 3, providing protection from activation of the cell death cycle that leads to apoptosis. In this process, CBD is providing protection for neurons.[20] CBD also decreases adenosine uptake by macrophages and microglial cells by blocking the equilibrative nucleoside transporter 1. This then causes the activation of adenosine A2A receptors, creating an immunosuppressive action on the microglia and the macrophages and a decrease in TNF-alpha.[80-83] The decrease in TNF-alpha reduces both oxidative and nitrosantive stress, as well as the mitochondrial superoxide generation induced by high glucose. There is a further reduction in production of the NF-kB protein in the endothelial cells, reduced nitro tyrosine formation, and prevention of the expression of iNOS. CBD also prevents the expression of the adhesion molecules ICAM-1 (an intercellular adhesion molecule) and VCAM-1 (a vascular cell adhesion molecule) by the endothelial cells; by preventing the expression of these compounds, CBD helps limit new inflammatory-promoting cells from entering into the tissues.[83]

CBD also attenuates dopamine depletion, accomplished by a reduction of tyrosine hydroxylase deficits[85] and indicative of a degree of narrow degeneration. With a newer perspective, we can measure the correlation between N-acetyl aspartate and total creatinine. When this ratio is elevated, there is increased neurogenesis and synaptogenesis,[85] and a decrease in copper-zinc superoxide dismutase. This enzyme is an endogenous defense against oxidative stress. CBD has also been shown to reduce striatal atrophy.

Several factors indicate an increased risk for the development of Parkinson's disease. There is some genetic susceptibility, seen through alpha-synuclein that has a tendency to fold; when it folds it is less likely to be broken down and removed. Usually, conformational plasticity is greater, and these proteins can stay single, fold, or form into monomeric or oligomeric compounds. With the more complex folding, they become more stimulating for the production of problematic compounds. The complex compounds are more likely to form into amyloidogenic filaments that cause more cell damage.[86]

These filaments are highly expressed in mammalian brains, and are increased in presynaptic nerve terminals and associated with cell membranes and the secular structures.[87] They are also associated with membrane microdomains-lipid rafts; these are used for synaptic localization[88] and assist in synaptic vesicle recycling and dopamine neurotransmission.[89] In synaptic vesicle recycling, it is shown that alpha-synuclein support the function in recycling and dopamine neurotransmission.[90] CBD also binds to and blocks the activity of phospholipase D (PLD).[91]

This helps regulate lipid metabolism by protecting lipid droplets from hydrolysis.[92] CBD helps to regulate the size of presynaptic vesicle pools[93] and alpha-synuclein. The CBD also helps to regulate the size of synaptic vesicles, which store and recycle neurotransmitters. They also assist in recycling, particularly neurotransmitter dopamine, for storage, release, and recycling.

The alpha-synuclein oligomers are precursors for higher-order aggregates, which are amyloid-like fibrils referred to in Parkinson's disease as filamentous structures in Lewy bodies and Lewy neuritis.[94] The monomers can form annular fibrils or combine into protofibrils to form Lewy bodies.[84,95] Similar to pore-forming bacterial toxins, annular fibrils can open pores into the cells.[96] These protofibrils may cause more cell membrane permeability; and the catecholamines, especially dopamine, can react with alpha-synuclein to form covalent bonds. There can be a slow conversion of protofibrils to fibrils,[97] and protofibrils may be cytotoxic.[98] The cytotoxicity seen with fibrils and inclusion bodies[99-101] promotes the formation of more alpha-synuclein.[101-195]

The increased production of alpha-synuclein starts to affect mitochondrial complex 1, acting as an inhibitor—along with rotenone and paraquat—and creating more oxidative and nitrosative stress.[106] This leads to more oxidative damage and selective tyrosine nitration of the alpha-synuclein in Parkinson's disease.[107] The tyrosine nitration of alpha-synuclein promotes further fibril formation of unmodified alpha-synuclein. This leads to a decreased rate of degradation of the 20S proteasome and cysteine protease calpain 1.[108]

An increase of alpha-synuclein in the human substantia nigra happens with age, and this process needs stabilization to prevent accumulation and to reduce oxidative stress. Without intervention, the oxidative stress can lead to protein modifications.

The major damage in Parkinson's disease is from oxidative stress, hyperexcitability, and reduced energy production from mitochondrial damage. These have been shown to be addressed by cannabinoids, especially CBD. The protection is from CBD's direct effect on neurons and its effect on the glial cells. It is through the use of cannabinoids that we may see advances made in the treatment of Parkinson's disease. It has been shown that the cannabinoids can prevent damage to the dopaminergic neurons, or even their death.

X

Huntington's Disease

Huntington's disease is an inherited neurodegenerative disorder. The normal gene for huntingtin protein is present but when you have the disease you have additional material in the form of repeats of CAG; the more of the repeats you have, the more severe the problem. Called the huntingtin gene (HTT), in the genetic coding C=cytosine, A=adenine, and G=guanine. There is an elongated stretch of glutamine near the NH2 terminus of the protein,[2] and the 6 through 35 repetitions of this segment are very unstable with a tendency to expand from one generation to the next.[19,20] The absolute numbers of this expansion affect the severity and progression of Huntington's disease. Those with 40 or more CAG repeats will exhibit Huntington's disease.[2] When there are 60 or more, the disease develops in childhood or during the juvenile period.[2, 21, 22]

A mutation in the huntingtin protein is the triggering event for the development of Huntington's disease. These mutated proteins cause toxic functions and will affect some specific subpopulations of neurons in the stratum, leading to chorea. In the cerebral cortex, they create cognitive deficiencies and lead to dementia. These mutated proteins create brain neurodegeneration leading to a loss of efferent medium spiny neurons. In the stratum, GABAergic neurons are affected by the mutated proteins located in the caudate nucleus, putamen, and medium-sized spiny neurons. Atrophy and loss of cells is prominent in the caudate and putamen.[3,9]

In 1985, Dr. J. P. Vonsattel created a grading system based on neuronal location and severity of neuronal loss. Four classes are based on the basal ganglia,[3] with classes three and four seeing the broadest effects. In the cerebral cortex, layers three, five, and six are affected, with additional ones noted in the globus pallidus, thalamus, subthalamic nuclei, substantia nigra, white matter, cerebellum,[9] and hypothalamus.[10, 11]

Widespread neurodegeneration also involves cortical structures.[4-6] The mutation leads to an impairment of the ability of normal huntingtin protein to perform its normal and fundamental activities. These activities support the survival and functioning of the neurons that degenerate within the CNS.[7,8] These can produce cognitive deficits in attention, working memory, and executive function.[12-15] Large reductions in the brain's volume occur[4, 16] before any symptoms are noted from the abnormalities in the cortex. Adult onset usually occurs between 35 and 50 years of age. In cases of juvenile onset, it will occur before 20 years of age with an approximate 10 percent paternal transmission.[17, 18] Symptoms include personality changes, generalized motor dysfunctions, and cognitive decline.

The normal function of huntingtin protein contributes to polyQ forms that bind to transcription factors.[25] Through these factors, this protein supports cell longevity and energy status and associates with mitochondria, golgi, and the endoplasmic reticulum.[26,27] It can also associate in the nucleus,[29] where it helps to modulate calcium homeostasis.[27] The mutant huntingtin protein aggregates in neurons, both intracellular and intranuclear. This can affect the cells' autonomous actions[23] and cell-to-cell interactions.[24] The process can lead to activation of NMDA receptors, creating excess excitation.

Huntington protein is highly expressed in cortical pyramidal neurons of layers 3 and 5. These neurons project to striatal neurons.[28] It associates with vesicular structures within the indissoluble compartments and microtubules.[30] Its function here is to promote the production of BDNF and to transport it along microtubules.[32] The protein also helps support the cytoskeleton and participates in morphogenesis, supports endocytosis and exocytosis, and participates in modulating cell apoptosis. It helps to regulate synaptic activity, as multiple repeats in the protein can impair synaptic transmission. It participates in the modulation of gene transcription[25, 31] and helps to regulate cerebral spinal fluid.[33] It is also critical in participating in the modulation of mitochondrial function.

With the loss of wild-type (normal) huntingtin protein, the neurons' ability to survive is reduced, as is the ability to remove the toxic effects created by the mutant protein.[36] Wild-type huntingtin protein reduces the toxicity of the mutant huntingtin protein.[37] There is a reduction in the production of BDNF gene transcription,[38] which leads to a loss of BDNF that is provided to the striatal neurons (medial spinal neurons, or MSNs).

The BDNF protein is produced in the cortex and moved in an an1terograde transport along the cortical striatal tract to the MSNs.[39] The BDNF is needed for nerve cell growth and survival, and the mutant huntingtin protein reduces its production.[40] The repressor element-1 transcription factor/neuron restrictive silencer factor (REST/NRSE) begins to accumulate in the nucleus, which reduces the transcription of BDNF.[8] There is also a reduction in BDNF vesicle transport[32] that leads to reduction in the MSN soma size, and the development of fewer dendritic spines and thinner dendrites.[41]

During this process, excitotoxicity and a dysfunction in neuronal interactions and circuits are increased, also noted in the cortical striatal synapses. Excess glutamate receptor activation leads to increased glutamate release from the cortical afferents that is further aggravated by reduced glial cell uptake. We see a loss of NMDARs, [42] and increased sensitivity in the remaining ones.[45]

The presence of mutant huntingtin protein increases the sensitivity of the neurons to excitement[1] and leads to impaired synaptic plasticity,[43] which is necessary for modulation and adaptation to change. There is also a loss of connectivity between the cortex and stratum,[44] and dysregulation of calcium storage in the mitochondria, creating mitochondrial swelling. This is accentuated by mutant huntingtin protein, which affects transition pores[47] and leads to a release of cytochrome c and apoptotis-inducing factor (AIF).[46]

The neurotransmitter system contributes to the cortical striatal connections. Neuron activity can affect glutamate release, and in Huntington's disease both adenosine A2A receptors and input to these receptors is noted with an increase in receptor density in the striatum. There is also increased adenylyl cyclase activity, further increasing excitotoxicity.[49,50] Cannabinoid receptors[51] and, in particular, CB1 receptors, can increase glutamate release. This can add to an increase in excitotoxicity. Dopamine can directly control glutamate release through D2 receptors, and these may stimulate glutamate release.[48] There is a parallel between dopamine and glutamine activity. It has been shown that dopamine receptor antagonists improve the symptoms of Huntington's disease.[1]

Huntingtin protein is cleaved by caspases 1, 2, 3, and 7. Preventing these cleavages from occurring helps decrease the symptoms of Huntington's disease and prolongs the time before neuronal inclusions begin.[52] Caspase 6 cleavage is very toxic.[53] This is a crucial event in the disease process,[1, 53] and the first step leading to multiple caspase activations.[1, 53] This leads to the formation of aggregates of the polyQ expansions.[54-57]

Aggregates are correlated with cell death,[58, 59] and there is greater toxicity when these are localized in the nucleus.[60] This leads to the sequestration of transcriptional regulators.[61, 62] The ubiquitin-proteasome system (UPS) cannot break down the mutant huntingtin protein.[63-65] Aggregates may be formed to protect against the toxic fragment.[66, 67] The aggregates stimulate the autophagy and help process and clear the mutant protein.[68] The aggregates are placed in autophagosomes or autophagic vacuoles. These then merged with lysosomes, resulting in a degradation of the contents. This process protects cells from death.[69]

Mutant huntingtin protein can bind directly to the mitochondria themselves,[47] contributing to dysfunction and leading directly to altered metabolic activity and altered calcium-induced permeability.[71] The consequent release of cytochrome[47] leads to reduced efficiency and energy production in the mitochondria. Altered motility[70] is seen with reduced mitochondrial membrane potential.[71] The mitochondria themselves also become the product of and a target for ROS.[72]

Dysfunction of lipid metabolism and cholesterol is precipitated by a reduction in transcription of cholesterol biosynthetic pathways.[73] This process affects cell membranes, making them more susceptible to ROS. This is complicated by malfunction in membrane trafficking and a dysregulation of myelin formation. All of these have a tremendous impact on synaptogenesis.[1, 74] The mutant huntingtin protein binds directly to DNA and prevents the transcription of some genes.[75] There is a hypoacetylation of H3 histones, down-regulating some genes.[76]

Included in the major changes seen in Huntington's disease is a conformational change in the protein from all the poly-glutamine additions. This affects protein-to-protein interactions, the formation of fragments, the formation of aggregates, and the resistance of the mutant protein to breakdown. These combine to lead to transcriptional dysregulation and a reduction in neuronal survival because of reduced BDNF. There is also mitochondrial dysfunction relating to complex II deficiency and calcium imbalance and an interruption in mitochondrial membrane integrity. These issues are further complicated by increasing excitotoxicity, oxidative stress, and glial activation. The glial activation includes astrocytosis, increasing numbers of reactive microglial and local inflammation, which spreads.

CBD can help reduce the hyperkinetic symptoms of Alzheimer's[77] and can also protect striatal neurons from death. It offers protection and provides neuroregenerative properties.[78, 79] A correlation with the down-regulation in the neurons is a loss of CB1 receptors in the stratum, this leads to a selective destruction of medium-spiny GABAergic neurons.[80, 81] CBD helps control the release of glutamate,[88] which occurs in the early phases of Huntington's disease. Inhibition of FAAH increases the stimulation of CB1 receptors.[91] During the inflammation and neurodegeneration, there is an up-regulation of CB2 receptors in glial cells in response to the damage.

The activated astrocytes influenced by CBD have enhanced trophic support.[79,82] Microglia activated[78,79,83] through stimulation of the CB2 receptors reduces the astrocytes' cytotoxicity and thereby reduce their production of free radicals and proinflammatory activities.[79,82] CBD enhances cell survival,[84,85] provides neuroprotection,[92,93] and helps to normalize glutamate homeostasis.[95,96] CBD helps to reduce oxidative stress[97,98] and reduces or attenuates glial activation. It also helps to reduce local inflammatory events[99, 100] and helps modulate the effect on genes.[101] This genetic intervention helps reduce the stress response and inflammation.

CBD also provides protection and support for the mitochondria. It helps to reduce oxidative stress with its two hydroxyl groups[94] and also helps to restore normal balance, reducing oxidative stress.[102] Through these activities, CBD works to enhance neuronal survival and normal intracellular mechanisms that support the endogenous antioxidant enzymes and to control the oxidative stress that is generated.[91] This is controlled through CBD's activity with transcription factors, and nuclear factor-erythroid 2-related factor (nrf-2). Through this mechanism, CBD's activity leads to an increase in transcription factors that can respond to oxidative stress.[102]

CBD also provides calcium (Ca2+) modulation within the mitochondria,[87] accomplished through control of TRPA1 calcium channels, and TRPV1 and TRPV2 receptors.[91] These functions are independent of cannabinoid receptors and some of it is independent of TRPVI receptors.[87] Some of these activities are also independent of the adenosine A2A receptors[87] that help scavenge free radicals.[82]

CBD also helps induce the reduction in proinflammatory cytokines such as IL-2 and TNF-alpha.[89] It increases the production of BDNF, which is necessary for neuronal survival.[90] Some of the anti-inflammatory activities are independent of CB2 receptors, including control of microglial cell migration,[103] the control of proinflammatory cytokines,[104] and the inhibitory control of NFkB signaling.

CBD controls the genes regulated by inducible nitric oxide synthase (iNOS).[104,105] It also helps to reduce the phosphorylation of kinases, controls transcription factors, and prevents translocation of the molecules into the nucleus, thereby preventing expression of pro-inflammatory genes.[105] CBD further binds the nuclear receptor PPAR-gamma,[107] which acts to antagonize the action of NFkB. This activity reduces proinflammatory enzymes, such as iNOS, ox-2, cytokines, and metalloproteinases.[107]

From this information, it is easy to deduce that CBD can have a pivotal role in the treatment of Huntington's disease. The issues are going to be the recognition of early signs of the disease and when the administration of CBD would be most benefitial. The action of this phytocannabinoid can help address all the issues that are created during the process and evolution of Huntington's disease. From a theoretical point, nothing but benefit that can be derived from the use of CBD in the treatment of Huntington's disease. It is my hope that the studies will be done and that, if this theory is correct, many people will benefit from this intervention.

XI

Multiple Sclerosis

Multiple sclerosis is a chronic inflammatory disorder of the CNS, including the brain, spinal cord, and optic nerves.[2] Sclerosis refers to scarring,[1] the result of the destruction of the myelin sheath that is the wrapping around the nerves. There are some factors that have been considered to predispose some people to the development of multiple sclerosis,[23] including some genetic predispositions, some viral infections, and a predisposition or development of autoimmunity. In multiple sclerosis, considered an autoimmune disease, myelin is destroyed.[4] The underlying nerve tissue itself can be damaged or destroyed when the immune system attacks its own body's tissue.[1] One of the biggest issues in this disease is the movement of leukocytes across the blood-brain barrier; when they cross the barrier, they become activated and begin to produce proinflammatory cytokines and cause the escalation of the inflammation in the brain.[24]

Multiple sclerosis takes several forms,[2] and the most commonly used classification for the forms is empirical (derived from experimentation). The first and most common form is relapsing-remitting multiple sclerosis (RRMS).[2] Symptoms can appear for days to weeks and then resolve spontaneously. The bouts reoccur approximately every one to two years. Inflammatory lesions develop and continue to do so even during symptom-free periods. The second form is secondary progressive multiple sclerosis (SPMS). In this form, two preexisting neurological deficits worsen over time and relapses occur in the end stages. The third form is primarily progressive multiple sclerosis (PPMS)[3] This form is characterized by a gradual neurological progression from the onset, with fewer abnormalities appearing on brain magnetic resonance imaging (MRI). It is also less responsive to standard therapies. The fourth form is progressive relapsing multiple sclerosis (PRMS). In this form neurologic function worsens gradually, with subsequent superimposed relapses. This may be a variant of SPMS, with the suggestion that the initial relapses were unrecognized or clinically silent. Some speculate that relapses are forgotten by the person.

Multiple sclerosis usually begins between the ages of 20 and 40 years.[1] It is usually seen with recurrent bouts of central nervous inflammation[2] and damage to the myelin sheath around axons (known as demyelination). The damage may even affect the axons themselves.[5] In demyelinating lesions, there are more than 11,000 transected axons per cubic millimeter; the normal brain has fewer than 1/ per cubic millimeter.[2] Transected neurons can no longer transmit information; this damage is created from the immune system activation and is part of the damage in multiple sclerosis.

Severe demyelination can occur, and the number of axons and oligodendrocytes can decrease. The immune system responds against unknown CNS antigens.[2] The inflammation that occurs can be generated from T-cell mediated or T-cell-plus mediated autoimmune responses. These are two specific types of T-cells that are found associated with autoimmune disease. One of the primary disorders affects the oligondendrocytes, which produce the myelin.[4]

Cortical demyelination plays a critical role in multiple sclerosis pathogenesis and cognitive dysfunction. These may occur early in the disease.[6] Oligodendrocytes progenitor cells capable of remyelination have been observed in the white-matter plaques.[7]

The diagnosis of multiple sclerosis has no specific diagnostic criteria[2] but is instead based upon clinical history, laboratory findings, and imaging results. In 1965 the Schumacher criteria for the diagnosis of multiple sclerosis established, purely on the basis of clinical findings: there must be CNS lesions disseminated in space and time, and alternative diagnoses must be eliminated.[8] The McDonald criteria were formed to bring more relevant MRI information for the basis of diagnosis and treatment. Originally established in 2001, they were revised in 2005 and again in 2010. With these criteria, diagnosis is made on the basis of clinical characteristics alone or in combination with MRI features.[9] The conventional therapies for multiple sclerosis include methylprednisolone (for acute relapses), interferon-beta, and other medications.

Several factors have been shown to predispose people to multiple sclerosis. One study showed that low vitamin D level predisposes to multiple sclerosis.[1] Another study showed people who are smokers are more likely to get multiple sclerosis.[1]

The symptoms seen in multiple sclerosis patients depend on the nerves that are attacked;[1] therefore, not everyone will have the same symptoms. Some people will display sensory nerve symptoms because those are the nerves that are demyelinating. Others will show motor symptoms because those neurons are affected. And in some people, the spine is affected because of demyelination in the spine, with symptoms that can present either unilaterally or bilaterally.[1]

Some of the earliest symptoms can be tingling, numbness, pain, burning, or itching. These symptoms may occur in the arms, legs, trunk, or face, depending on which nerves are affected. Some people even have a reduced sense of touch. Other more dramatic symptoms can be changes in the visual field; nystagmus (involuntary, rapid eye movement), a symptom that may be either transitory or progressively evolve; double vision; and even a complete loss of vision. Other symptoms include weakness, spasticity, and slurring of speech.

The typical picture of multiple sclerosis is that of remissions when symptoms reduce, and it is felt that the disease is reducing its rate of attack. This can be followed by relapses, where new symptoms or evolving symptoms occur as the disease becomes active again. However, in some of the newer studies, it is noted that the demyelination is continuing, even in periods that appear to be in remission.[3,4,6]

Cannabinoids are useful in the treatment of multiple sclerosis. They can help improve motor function, reduce activated microglia, and promote remyelination of the spinal cord.[10, 12] These compounds provide treatment beyond just symptomatic relief of pain and motor impairment.

With cannabinoid therapy, pain is reduced, followed by a reduction in spasticity, rigidity, and tremor.[11] Viral models of multiple sclerosis show a reduction of spasticity and tremor,[11] produced through cannabinoid receptor agonists THC and Win55,212-2[12], which is a synthetic compound that acts to stimulate cannabinoid CB1 receptors. However, there are also activities that are independent of cannabinoid receptors, using neither CB1 nor CB2 receptors. There appears to be a "CB2-like" receptor reacts with an endogenous cannabinoid palmitoylethanolamide. This activity can be blocked by CB2 receptor antagonists.[13-15]

It has been shown that spasticity can be reduced by blocking both the endocannabinoid membrane transporter and the hydrolysis of the naturally occurring cannabinoids.[16] CBD can also reduce microglial activation, leading to reduced inflammation.[16] The action of CBD blocks the membrane transporter, thereby increasing the amount of endogenous cannabinoid that is available to help reduce pain and spasticity.

CBD further acts as an antioxidant because of its biochemistry and its modification and modulation of cell signaling.[18] Through the modulation of cell signaling, it reduces the self-sustaining cycles of inflammation and oxidative stress. These CBD activities are carried out through noncannabinoid receptors. CBD acts as a competitive inhibitor of adenosine uptake in both macrophages and microgial cells. Activation of A2A adenosine receptors[19] has an immunosuppressive effect on these cells. It decreases the amount of TNF-alpha that is produced by the microglial cells and is proinflammatory.

CBD acts to reduce oxidative and nitrosative stress.[18] This is accomplished by reducing super oxide generation and blocking the activation of NF-kB, which would lead to the production of free radicals. It further blocks both the activation of iNOS and the proinflammatory signaling from activated microglial cells.[20] CBD decreases the production of NF-kB and prevents the activation of a signal transducer and activator of transcription (STAT), STAT-1, which are both inflammatory. It also increases the anti-inflammatory signaling through the STAT-3 pathway.

Neuropathic pain is believed to be derived from microglial activation in the spinal cord and brain. It continues and is aggravated by the proinflammatory cytokines that are produced, including interleukin-1 beta, IL-6, and TNF-alpha. When activated, these microglia generate more oxygen species and intiation factors that tend to continue the cycle.[21]

CBD helps control nociceptive inputs to the CNS, and, when these are blocked, neuropathic pain is reduced.[22] CBD also decreases the expression of VCAM-1. VCAM-1 is an adhesion molecule, when you reduce its production then you reduce the number of monocytes and lymphocytes coming into the inflammed area. This helps to reduce further expansion of inflammation. These cells are part of the ongoing cycle of inflammation and neurodegeneration. CBD reduces the up-regulation of chemokines, such as CCL2 and CCL5. These compounds are produced from astrocytes and perpetuate the up-regulation of inflammation neurodegeneration. One of the most powerful effects of CBD is that it restricts immune-cell transmigration into the CNS.

In the TMEX-viral model of multiple sclerosis,[23] early treatment with CBD in the acute phase had broad application in controlling the disease. It prevented the development of motor abnormalities and the progression to a chronic phase. It also reduced microglia activation, thereby reducing inflammation, demyelination, and axonal loss. In the model of multiple sclerosis, CBD was also shown to decrease the production of proinflammatory cytokines IL-1 beta, TNF-alpha, IL-2, IL-6, IL-12, and IFN-gamma. CBD was shown to induce cell proliferation in the microglial cells;[28] it was further shown that it could modulate migration of the cells that create inflammation in the CNS, thereby reducing the number of new immune cells recruited to propagate the inflammatory process. CBD reduces antigen presentation and that will reduce the number of activated proinflammatory cells. It also controls the number of new immune cells which are coming into the area. By these two mechanisms CBD helps reduce inflammation and damage to neurons.

CDB decreased adenosine uptake through A2A receptors, leading to a reduced release of VCAM-1.[25] When this release is reduced, the adhesion of lymphocytes to the endothelial cells is lessened, enabling the blood-brain barrier to stay intact and reducing the effect of high glucose on the endothelial cells, thereby reducing inflammation.[23,25] This process reduces the leukocyte infiltration, further decreasing chemokine production,[26] and reducing symptoms.

This is part of the immune modulation that is provided by CBD.[23] It limits the recruitment of lymphocytes to the inflamed site and modulates the activity of astrocytes and microglial cells.[29] It also produces anti-inflammatory effects through its action on A2A receptors that both block and stop effects[23] on endothelial cells.

CBD will protect oligodendrocyte progenitor cells,[30] the cells that produce myelin, by preventing their destruction and enabling the body with a pathway to produce more myelin. The loss of oligodendrocytes is the hallmark of multiple sclerosis. CBD works to prevent damage from oxidative stress by protecting mitochondria and preventing damage to the endoplasmic reticulum. CBD has also been shown to replace the oligodendrocytes that are destroyed by the process of neuroinflammation.[31] When the endoplasmic reticulum is stressed, the stress response will produce serine/threonine kinase (PKR), and eIF-2 alpha, which creates an increase in phosphorylation. This phosphorylation increase promotes the processing and production of protein in response to stress. When these are triggered, the integrity of the endoplasmic reticulum is disrupted, and apoptosis in the oligodendrocytes is induced.

There is some speculation from the MS Microbiome Consortium, a group of scientists looking into possible causes of multiple sclerosis,[32] that noted abnormal bacteria in the microbiome of multiple sclerosis patients that can alter immune function. There is an increase in Methanobrevibacteriaceae flora present in people with multiple sclerosis. This flora can cause an increase in immune activity and is greatly increased in multiple sclerosis patients with a depletion of bacteria that can suppress immune function.

As with other diseases, multiple sclerosis appears to have multiple mechanisms, triggers, predisposing factors, and possible explanations for the disease. From the research that has been done, CBD appears to be effective in treating the disease, especially when added early in the disease process. It provides activity through both cannabinoid and noncannabinoid receptors, and it is through this diversity that CBD can have a broad application for multiple sclerosis in treating symptoms such as pain, spasticity, and tremors. The greater application is in the modulation of oxidative stress and neurodegeneration, and it is in these areas that no present treatment exists that can provide those affects.

XII

Pain

Pain is a very complicated subject, made more so because of its subjectivity. When someone is in pain, we do not really know how much pain they feel, nor the severity or how long it has lasted. Pain is something that's been with us since the beginning of time, and it is something that we have struggled to effectively treat. Today we have many modalities and medications that we use to treat pain; unfortunately, many of these are addictive.

A whole segment of society is addicted to pain medications today, partially because we are only guessing at the nature of the pain. Because of the subjectivity and difficulty of knowing what each person is feeling, choosing the right treatment becomes even more difficult. Even pain scales are very subjective, as people find it difficult to express exactly what they are sensing and feeling. This, too, makes treatment difficult.

There are many types of pain, but we are mainly going to discuss two: inflammatory and neuropathic pain.[7,8,24] The underlying mechanisms of these types of pain differ. Neuropathic pain[48] is frequently chronic, and the neurons in the brain or the peripheral nervous system become hypersensitized. These neurons then generate abnormal or prolonged impulses that increase the sensitivity to pain. Other types of pain include diabetic and cancer neuropathy, postherpetic neuralgia, brachial plexus lesions, fibromyalgia, and multiple sclerosis. Research shows that

40 percent of cancer patients have neuropathic-created pain.[57] Similar receptors are used to process noxious stimuli, including mechanical, thermal, and chemical.

The use of cannabis has a very long history as a pain reliever.[9,10] Its first recorded use was more than 5,000 years ago in Chinese society, when the Chinese physician Hoa-Gho described the use of cannabis for surgical anesthesia. Between 315 and 392 CE, cannabis was used in ancient Israel for childbirth.

Present treatment for pain is only effective in approximately 50 percent of patients.[48] Today, the most commonly prescribed medications for significant pain are opioids. These compounds are addictive. Much of the recent research has shown the cannabinoids are more effective and use a different mechanism,[54] as the cannabinoid receptors are on afferent myelinated A fibers. Pain transmission is carried through these fibers,[56] and, since there are fewer mu-opioid receptors, the opioids are less efficient in controlling the pain at the spinal-cord level.

Cannabinoids selectively suppress noxious stimuli in the spinal and thalamic nocio neurons.[11-15] These help provide antinocioceptive effects.[1-4] In animal models of nocioceptive or different types of noxious symptom stimuli, there have been many studies that show that cannabinoids are equal in efficacy and potency to opiates.[5] Systemic administration of cannabinoids suppresses behavioral reactions to acute noxious stimuli and further reduces inflammatory pain and pain from nerve injury.

Much of this has been shown to be through CB1 receptors, helping to suppress nociceptive transmission.[5] The receptors also act to decrease the perception of pain.[48] When pain is present, there is an up-regulation of CB2 receptors at the sites of nociceptive processing. There is also an induction of CB2 receptors when neuropathic pain is present.[65,66]

Exogenous cannabinoids can act at peripheral, spinal, and superspinal levels,[5] and they are not limited to one point of activity. The inhibition of the enzymes FAAH and monoacyl glycerol lipase (MGL) can also inhibit the production of nocioception.[6] FAAH breaks down the endogenous cannabinoid anandamide that is active at CB1 receptors. Monoacylglycerol is the enzyme that breaks down arachidonyl glycerol (2-AG) that is active at CB2 receptors. When either of these two compounds are increased, they can decrease nocioception.

Many of the cannabinoids have a central action in the brain; some of the studies that have been done have injected these compounds into the intracerebral ventricular system. In these studies, the central action of these compounds reduced pain sensitivity. They were found to be active in the dorsal lateral periaquaductal gray,[49] the dorsal raphe nucleus, the rostral ventral medulla, the amygdala, and the lateral posterior and submedius regions of the thalamus. This is the area of input from a spinal thalamic pathway[48] associated with pain. They are also active at the superior colliculus and noradrenergic nucleus A5.[16-18] All of these are central areas involved with the processing of pain. The descending adrenergic system is active in mediating peripheral effects of pain.[19, 26]

When CB1 receptors are activated, the result is a mixture of pain relief and some psychotropic effects. This is one of the limiting factors of using CB1 receptor agonists. Since these are the receptors that modulate the psychotropic activity, this can limit the dosage range of the agonists.

Another place where the cannabinoids work is at the spinal level, where they decrease the spinal reflexes to noxious stimuli.[21] The CB1 receptors in the spine inhibit C fibers and A-delta fibers.[22] Research also shows an interaction between cannabinoid and opiate receptors. THC has been shown to increase the effectiveness of morphine, and, with this increase in effectiveness, a reduced dose can be used to control the pain. THC has been shown to act at kappa and delta opioid receptors[48] whose stimulation acts synergistically with opiates.[62]

In the periphery, these compounds also work to control inflammation. The CB1 receptors decreased input from pain sensors. CB1 and CB2 agonists act in the periphery to decrease nocioception[24] and, through this decrease, the input and perception of pain. CB2 receptors in the periphery help reduce nocioception. These receptors have no psychotropic effects,[24] but they act against both acute and persistent pain.[25-29] They help to inhibit the release of proinflammatory cytokines and proinflammatory factors that affect nociceptive nerve terminals. They also stimulate mu-opioid receptors[48] and act to stimulate the release of the endogenous opioid beta-endorphins.[48-50]

CB2 receptors are on peripheral nerve fibers[30] and on the spinal cord.[63] Microglial activation is reduced through these CB2 receptors, and the immune response of the microglial cells contributes to neuropathic pain.[67-70]

When 5 mg of delta-9-THC was administered in a study, it decreased the ability to distinguish pain.[31] In another study 0.022-0.044 mg per kilogram (kg) of delta-9-THC was given intravenously and was shown to increase the pain threshold.[32]

Acute pain is typically managed with opioids today; however, these do not work effectively when the pain is related to nerve injury.[48] THC, on the other hand, is antinociceptive even after nerve injury.[54] Cannabinoids have also been shown to be effective in alleviating what is referred to as intractable pain syndrome.[48]

Chronic pain differs from acute pain because of neural changes that occur within the affected fibers that tend to prolong the noxious stimuli.[24] Allodynia, a decreased pain threshold, occurs with a heightening of the painful threshold of the noxious stimuli referred to as hyperalgesia. This process is also referred to as the wind-up phenomenon.[48] Many studies show that cannabinoids are more effective than opioids at controlling this problem.

In several cancer pain studies where the cancer pain was felt to be moderately intense,[33-35] 20 mg of THC was equivalent to 120 mg of codeine. This was also seen with the compound Sativex (nabiximol) when used in animal studies using an animal model of cancer.[64] In a randomized placebo-controlled, graded-dose study, this compound reduced pain and improved sleep. The dosages were between 1 and 4 sprays per day or 6 and 10 sprays per day. The lower number of sprays produced the least side effects and the same efficacy.

In a study of multiple sclerosis that presented with neuropathic pain,[36] a dose of 10 mg per day decreased the intensity of pain and provided pain relief and improvement on a quality-of-life scale. Participants showed no changes in their functional ability. Significant muscle spasms often accompany multiple sclerosis, and studies indicate here as well that cannabis reduces the spasms. In addition, cannabis has been shown to halt the progression of multiple sclerosis, reducing neuropathic pain and correcting sleep disturbances.[55]

Neuropathic pain in multiple sclerosis is believed to begin from an autoimmune encephalomyelitis.[73] Because of the issues with psychotropic side effects, CB1 receptor agonists have to be modulated.[24] These psychotropic effects limit the amount of CB1 receptor agonists that can be used; therefore, these compounds may not be completely effective for neuropathic pain or nerve injury pain.

CBD can help with this pain due to its interaction or agonism of 5-HT1A receptors.[69] CBD helps suppress the up-regulation of microglial cells. Research shows that cytokines produced by the microglia sensitize neurons.[74] It is also been shown that CBD is an antagonist of 5-HT-3A receptors, and that this activity helps with nociception and the control of emesis.

Cannabinoid receptors function through G protein coupled receptors[37-40] with multiple differences in the subtypes of G protein receptors. When stimulated, some of these will cause pain reduction without psychotropic activity. Stimulating these receptors also does not cause motor dysfunction. There are different types of G-protein coupled receptors, some when stimulated will reduce pain and provide no psychotropic activity. There activity will be controlled by their location, those in the basal ganglia and cerebellum will affect motor control. For analgesia it would be those located in the periaqueductal gray, rostral ventral medulla, spinal cord, and peripheral nerves that modulate pain.[41-43] It has been seen in some studies that stimulation of some cannabinoid receptors may provide different functions on the basis of the allosteric structure of the compound used. It is speculated that it is these modifications in the structure of the molecules that enable it to interact with different G protein subtypes.

Research studies show that FAAH degrades anandamide, 2-AG, and N-arachidonyldopamine (NADA).[40-45] When you block the activity of FAAH, this leads to an increase in analgesia.[46] When this occurs, there is an increase in anandamide, which is an agonist for CB1 receptors. This analgesia is seen in both acute and chronic pain and creates a blunted sensitivity to pain. Blocking the protein cellular transport mechanism also leads to an increase in anandamide and an increase in analgesia.

Some nonsteroidal anti-inflammatory drugs (NSAIDs) enhance CB1 receptor activity.[51] Indomethacin, and fluribuprofen both act to inhibit FAAH.[52] They also block cyclooxygenase-2 (COX-2) activity, which increases anandamide and 2-AG.[67] It is through these activities that these compounds provide some analgesia. The activity of COX-2[53] facilitates the inflammatory response and can increase neuronal death. Cyclooxygenase catabolizes anandamide and 2-AG. This leads to a reduction of analgesia and an increase in pain perception.

Migraines are a different kind of pain and are considered to be vasomotor headaches. This is based on their pulsatile nature, their presentation in crisis, their periodic occurrence, and, for many, a hemicranial distribution (occurs on only one side of the brain). They can be associated in some people with generalized sensorial hyperesthesia, some sensitivity to light or noise (or both), and, in some, nausea or vomiting (or both). When you look at the symptoms, several studies have shown that cannabis has antimigraine properties.[58] In several of the studies, cannabis was shown to have equal or better pain relief than the present medications used to treat migraine, ergotamine and aspirin.[59]

Diabetic peripheral neuropathy is also a form of neuropathic pain.[60] The microglia cells have a prominent role, yet cannabinoid receptors are present on some neurons and microglial cells. Studies have shown that, during the normal course of diabetes, when no treatment is enacted, microglial density increases around neurons. This is seen in the dorsal spinal cord and the thalamus. Phosphorylated p38MAPK is elevated, an indication of activation of microglial cells. In addition, a reduction of both CB1 receptors[71] and FAAH leads to an increase in endocannabinoids.[72]

CBD has been shown to attenuate the development of neuropathic pain. In a study of CBD dosages of 0.1 mg/kg, 1 mg/kg, and 2 mg/kg, the effects elicited by CBD were continued even after discontinuation of compound, and no modifications were made in the diabetic state. CBD can work and reduce peripheral neuropathy and neuropathic pain. When CB1 and CB2 receptor agonists were used, the antinociception was only present when they were given and did not last after they were stopped.

CBD suppresses both inflammatory and neuropathic pain.[61] It has an interaction with and stimulates glycine alpha-3 receptors, and it interacts with the S296 in the third transmembrane domain.

Active in the dorsal horn of the spinal cord, it also interacts with TRPV1 receptors[68] that assist with the spinal control of pain. It reduces the degradation of anandamide, which is a CB1 receptor agonist. It also helps reduce pain through its agonist of 5-HT1A receptors.[69]

XIII

Nausea and Vomiting

The emetic reflex, which consists of nausea, retching, and vomiting, is a protective reflex occurring in many animals in nature, with some exceptions. The nausea and vomiting reflexes are both interwoven and parallel. Experimental animals have shown us that they are not the same system and are controlled separately.[1,2]

Vomiting expels toxins from the upper gastrointestinal tract. Nausea and pain, on the other hand, are warning signs. Nausea usually results in the cessation of consumption of whatever it is you have eaten, and it causes an aversion to be developed in the future[1]. The vomiting center in the brain stem is called the dorsal vagal complex. Located in the medulla, it is made up of three particular areas: area postrema (AP), nucleus tractus solitarii (nucleus of the solitary tract, or NTS) and dorsal motor nucleus of the vagas (dmnX).

There are multiple types of input and processing of emetogenic stimuli.[1,3,16] These include visual, olfactory, and pain sensory inputs processed through the limbic system. The receptors and neurotransmitters for the system consist of GABA and its receptors (GABA-R), as well as the cannabinoids and their receptors, particularly the CB1 receptors.

Another input is visceral irritants, such as foods, medications, radiation, and cytotoxic drugs. These compounds provide input locally in the stomach and small intestines. From there, neurotransmitters and their receptors transmit the information to the brain stem and the higher centers in the CNS. The local input here can be from hydrogen ions (H+); D2 dopamine receptors; histamine, through H1 receptors; and serotonin, through specific 5-HT3 receptors. Cannabinoid input is through CB1 and CB2 receptors, and neurokinin or substance P input is through neurokinin-1 (NK1) receptors. Any of these activations from these compounds is then passed on to the chemoreceptor trigger zone. These inputs may also directly affect this zone.

The terminals of the area postrema has its own receptors and neurotransmitters. In this area, serotonin acts through 5-HT3 receptors, dopamine through D2 receptors, histamine though H1 receptors, neurokinin or substance P thorugh NK1 receptors, and cannabinoids through CB1 receptors. The information sent here is then passed on to the solitary track (also known as the nucleus tractus solitarius), which has its own receptors and neurotransmitters. Similar to the ones in the area postreme, they consist of serotonin working through 5-HT3 receptors, dopamine through D2 receptors, histamine through H1 receptors, neurokinin or substance P through NK1 receptors, and cannabinoids through CB1 receptors. The output signals from here are then transmitted to the DMNX.

The DMNX receives input from multiple areas: the solitary track, the chemoreceptor trigger zone, the stomach, and the small intestine. It also receives input from the limbic system and higher centers, an input that comes from anxiety, memory, anticipation, and dread. The receptors and neurotransmitters transmitting these impulses are limited to GABA and cannabinoids through CB1 receptors.

Input from the cerebellum comes from the vestibular system through GABA and from cannabinoids through CB1 receptors. Sensory input feeds into this area, which is made up of visual stimuli, olfactory input, and pain, making it both a complex and very subjective input and interpretation.

Because of memory, anticipation, and visual and olfactory input, even the environment can contain triggers that will set off nausea and vomiting, and due to these factors of anticipation and memory, it has become one of the hardest areas to control. Anticipation of pain and nausea has been the hardest area to relieve in cancer patients receiving chemotherapy.

In review, the brain stem's neurotransmitters and receptors include serotonin, dopamine, neurokinin or substance P, histamine, endorphins, acetylcholine, GABA, and cannabinoids. These are the compounds or mechanisms for vomiting. Nausea is more complicated and not so fully detailed.[17,18]

The serotonin 5-HT3 receptor antagonists work very well in acute vomiting. However, for nausea that is not acute, such as in delayed chemotherapy-induced nausea and vomiting (CINV) and refractory CINV (the nausea no longer responds to the medicines taken to prevent it), this remains a significant problem,[3] because these are not controlled by 5-HT3 antagonists.

Studies on experimental animals have shown that serotonin 5-HT3 antagonists, and substance P and neurokinin at NK1 receptor antagonists will control emesis. To control nausea, though, it seems that modulating the dopamine D2 receptors and cannabinoid receptors that affect CB1 activity is effective. Increasing anandamide, which acts through CB1 receptors, can also help control nausea. This has also been demonstrated by the use of FAAH enzyme blockers, which work by increasing the amount of anandamide that is available to act. It has been shown that these are all found in the areas of the brain that control emesis.[19]

Some of the most difficult issues with pain, nausea, and vomiting are around chemotherapy. These toxins are not removed from the body by vomiting and, as has been seen, are not self-limited.[2] The other very difficult problem is the anticipatory issues that occur after the first rounds of chemotherapy and before the next chemotherapy visit.[3] Researchers have shown that nausea is the more prominent problem, and not so much the vomiting. Acute nausea and vomiting can occur within minutes to hours of the chemotherapy administration. It will usually resolve within the first 24 hours, and the intensity peaks after 5 to 6 hours. The next form is delayed nausea and vomiting, which can develop more than 24 hours after the demonstration of the chemotherapy agent. It can peak at 48 to 72 hours and may last as long as 6 to 7 days.

Breakthrough nausea and vomiting occurs despite prophylactic treatments. It requires some form of rescue therapy, and it may be acute or delayed. Refractory nausea and vomiting occurs in chemotherapy cycles despite prophylaxis and may also be seen when rescue therapy fails in earlier cycles.

The first major step for the physician is to control the vomiting. The serotonin receptor subtype of 5-HT3 receptors is specific to this problem, and experimental research has shown that an antagonist for the 5-HT3 receptor can prevent acute retching and vomiting.[1,4-8]

The 5-HT3 antagonists have been combined with corticosteroid dexamethasone in human studies, demonstrating that this combination can reduce acute vomiting in 70 to 90 percent of patients.[2,9-15] This combination does not work, however, for delayed nausea and vomiting and has been shown to be ineffective for breakthrough, refractory, and anticipatory nausea and vomiting.

This is where researchers have shown that the cannabinoids are helpful. It is the CB1 receptor activity that helps to reduce emesis. This is been shown experimentally for delta-9-THC. In addition, CB1 agonists or inverse agonists will increase vomiting.[20]

Delta-9-THC works at receptors in the area postrema and the nucleus of the solitary tract,[20,22] blocking the serotonin 5-hydroxytryptophan (5-HTP) receptor. Lower doses act centrally, and higher doses of 10 mg/kg act peripherally.[22]

CB2 receptors in the brain stem can contribute to antiemesis. 2-AG will affect both CB2 and CB1 receptors and helps to prevent emesis.[24] FAAH inhibitors alone, or those added to anandamide, prevent emesis induced by morphine-6-glucuronide.[24,25] The research suggests that this happened through the CB1 receptors.

In research done on the ferret, some of this antiemesis was produced through TRPV1 receptors.[25] Also noted are the endocannabinoids anandamide and NADA, both active at CB1 and TRPV1 receptors.[26] This research has led to the discovery of other avenues and receptors through which our endocannabinoids function.

Research has also shown that our cannabinoid system interacts with other neurotransmitter systems, in particular the definite interaction with 5-HT system.[27] The cannabinoids interact with both CB1 and 5-HT3 receptor in the dorsal vagal complex.[28,29] Both anandamide and synthetic cannabinoids inhibit 5-HT3 receptors.[30] Delta-9-THC has been shown to inhibit 5-HT3A receptors,[31] an innovation that is noncompetitive and binds at an allosteric site on this receptor.[31] This inhibition is not through direct interaction with the receptor but from its interaction at a different site.

CBD is a special case with low affinity for both CB1 and CB2 receptors.[32] In a rat model for nausea, at a low dose of 5 mg/kg, it inhibits vomiting and anticipatory retching.[33-36] As with other studies of CBD, there is a biphasic activity, and at a high dose of 20 to 40 mg/kg, it will potentiate vomiting.[33,34] Doses up to 20 mg/kg had no effect on 2-AG-induced vomiting.[37] This activity was not through CB1 receptors. Agonists of 5-HT1A receptors reduced serotonin's availability,[30] suggesting that through this mechanism, CBD controls nausea and vomiting.

CBD at 5 mg/kg suppresses vomiting by blocking 5-HT1A receptor antagonists and reducing the rate of neuronal firing and the levels of forebrain serotonin.[39] CBD also appears to be an allosteric inhibition of 5-HT3 receptors.[40] CBD also inhibits the reuptake of an anandamide,[1] which provides CB1 receptor activation and was shown to inhibit the breakdown of anandamide, which further increases its level and activity.[1]

As we've said previously that nausea is more difficult to control.[41] Using 5-HT3A antagonist can stop emesis, but there will still be activity in area postrem.[42] In the studies done in rats, they do not vomit but have a series of reactions that are felt to be the equivalent of nausea,[16] including gaping, chin rubbing, and paw treading. This pattern is also seen in animals before they vomit.[43] When linked to a stimulus, this pattern is referred to as conditioned gaping. It has been shown that delta-9-THC prevents condition gaping from occurring,[44] because of blocking blocked by CB1 receptor antagonists or inverse agonists.[45,46] It is also been shown that, by preventing the breakdown of anandamide, this will also block conditioned gaping[47] because this is a CB1 receptor agonist.

Research also shows that CBD reduces nausea by a non-cannabinoid mechanism. A dose of 5 mg/kg works to block nausea. This activity is carried out by serotonin receptors in the somatodedritic area by 5-HT1A auto receptors that are located in the dorsal raphe nucleus. Nausea appears to be mediated by 5-HT receptors acting in the forebrain in an area of the insular cortex.[48]

Anticipatory nausea develops over the course of repeated chemotherapy.[49] Whenever an event recurs, it produces more nausea, vomiting, or both. This is best understood as a classic conditioning response.[16,50] Control of anticipatory nausea is best at the time of conditioning or at the time of re-exposure to the conditioned stimulus.[16] Giving 5-HT3 receptor antagonists at the time of chemotherapy can prevent the formation of anticipatory nausea.[16,49] In addition, studies have shown that delta-9-THC prevents conditioned retching[16] and conditioned gaping.

CBD has also been shown to prevent anticipatory nausea[16,35] at a dosage range of 1 to 5 mg/kg.[16,51] At this dose, it prevents conditioned gaping and retching. At doses of 5 to 10 mg/kg, it prevents conditioned retching, but at doses of 20 to 40 mg/kg, it increases vomiting.[1,46] Since CBD also inhibits FAAH enzyme activity, it elevates the level of anandamide[16,51] and will prevent conditioned gaping.

Neuromodulation that is effective in controlling emesis is through the serotonin 5-HT3A receptors and substance P and neurokinin at NK1 receptors.[3] In summary, the most effective neuromodulation to control nausea is through control of dopamine D2 receptors and cannabinoids at the CB1, CB2, and 5-HT1A receptors.[16]

XIV

Arthritis

The presence of arthritis implies that there is inflammation in one or more joints.[2] Symptoms can be joint pain, stiffness, tenderness, locking, and a crackling noise referred to as crepitus. When the joint is inflamed, it can be swollen from an effusion of fluid. Arthritis has many causes and forms, and most forms worsen with age. The two most common forms are osteoarthritis and rheumatoid arthritis.

Osteoarthritis[1] is the most common form of arthritis and affects the synovial joints.[25] Also referred to as degenerative arthritis, degenerative joint disease, and degradation of joints, the articular cartilage will be eroded and appear soft, frayed, and thinned. The arthritis is actually not limited to the joint and articular surfaces, as inflammation can extend down into the subchondral bone, the bone to which the cartilage is attached. It is seen mainly in weight-bearing joints, such as the knees and hips, but it has also been known to affect the hands, feet, and spine. While the exact cause of osteoarthritis is unknown, we believe that hereditary and developmental abnormalities can predispose a person to the disease. In some cases, there is evidence of metabolic disturbances and mechanical wear and tear on the joint itself.

Examination of the joint will show erosion of the cartilage, even to the extent that bony surfaces are exposed. Inflammation can spread into the adjacent bone. This erosion of cartilage and exposure of the bone leads to pain that in turn leads to reduced range of motion and then muscle atrophy and lax ligaments.[3] The leading cause of chronic disability in the United States,[4] more than 27 million people are affected with osteoarthritis.

Rheumatoid arthritis is a chronic, systemic inflammatory disorder[25] that can lead to deformed joints that are painful and have lost function. The joints themselves are warm and tender, with increased stiffness early in the morning. This arthritis most commonly affects hands, feet, and the cervical spine, but it can also affect shoulders and knees. Just as in osteoarthritis, the causes are not understood.[6] With rheumatoid arthritis, we see an inflammatory response of the synovium, the capsule around the joint. There is swelling of the synovial cells, an excess of synovial fluid, and, over time, the development of fibrous tissue in the synovium called the pannus. There is also an erosion of the underlying bone, and thinning and destruction of the cartilage.[6]

In rheumatoid arthritis, inflammation can also affect other organs,[7] such as the pericardium (the lining around the heart), the pleural (the lining around the lungs), and the whites of the eyes. There can also be subcutaneous manifestations of inflammation, referred to as nodular lesions.

Both forms of arthritis are involved with inflammation, which is at the core of the disease itself. The form and extent of the inflammation varies with the disease, but, in both types of arthritis, we see immune system activation as a prominent feature. Both also have the loss of articular cartilage. The loss of cartilage is mediated through several modalities.[9] Proinflammatory cytokines, such as IL-1, IL-6, and TNF-alpha are involved, [25] as well as chemokine IL-8, nitric oxide, and prostraglandin E2 (PGE-2). We also see proteases, one of which is metalloproteinase, and aggrecanases, such as disintegrin and metalloproteinase with thrombospondin (ADMATS)-4 and -5. It also involves some anti-inflammatory compounds, such as IL-10 and TGF-beta.[25] These are the components—cytokines, chemokines and proteases—that lead to the destruction of cartilage. It is through control of these that an intervention can stop and prevent cartilage demise. Once the destructive process begins, immune cells are recruited that then are activated, and the inflammation may spread down through the cartilage, causing destruction of the subchondral bone.

Cannabinoids have been shown to reduce inflammation and prevent cartilage destruction. They are also capable of reducing nociceptive or sensory processing of the pain and thus help to reduce the pain perception that is associated with arthritis.[25] Cannabinoid agonists prevent the production of IL-1A,[10] one of the most potent destructive compounds of the cartilage. IL-1A induces proteoglycans and collagen degradation. It blocks the production of PGE2 and its activity on the chondrocytes. The chondrocytes are the cells that build cartilage; they have both CB1 and CB2 receptors. These help inhibit the activation of NFkB, a transcription factor that can modulate inflammation and compounds related to nitric oxide production. The cannabinoid agonists inhibit the expression of iNOS, prevent COX-2 activity, and block the activation of NFkB. These compounds stop the breakdown of articular cartilage.

CBD has also been shown to block the progression of osteoarthritis and rheumatoid arthritis in both mouse and rat models.[11,15] In a murine study where a chemical is injected to cause an acute arthritis and in chronic relapsing collagen-induced arthritis CBD will reduce symptoms of both types. When the dose was given intraperitoneally (injected into the peritoneum), the optimal effective amount was 5 mg/kg per day. When the dose was given orally, the optimal effective dose was 25 mg/kg per day. Both lower and higher doses were tested, and none were as effective as these optimal doses.

The murine studies showed that CBD reduced the production of collagen specific antibodies, reduced IFN-gamma production, and caused the suppression of lymphocyte proliferation. This suppression of lymphocyte proliferation was a general one, as the stimuli that usually lead to proliferation caused by mitogens or chemicals were suppressed. Even specific antigens— lipopolysaccharides from gram negative bacteria—which usually cause activation, did not induce the proliferation. These are two of the main types of activation that can lead to inflammation and introduce lymphocyte proliferation and activation.

CBD was also shown to decrease TNF-alpha production and the production of reactive oxygen bursts. It was also shown to inhibit cytotoxic T-cell activity. It suppressed the function of macrophages and their ability to present antigens, thereby reducing the number of activated immunocytes and thus the amount of inflammation. CBD further helps to reduce inflammation by modulating the production of TNF. It helps to reduce the production of IL-1 and IFN-gamma. Studies indicated that CBD further reduced the amount of a chemokine, IL-8, that was produced by B cells. These results were not strain specific.[11,15]

Studies also noted that in the acute form of arthritis, the mice treated with CBD had complete resolution. Those with the chronic form did not have complete resolution but did have a reduction in joint damage by 70+ percent. These studies clearly indicate that there is a dose-dependent suppression of both arthritis and joint damage with CBD.[11,12] Part of this activity is through immunosuppression, which leads to a shift away from T-helper 1 response, considered an inflammatory response. Part of the anti-inflammatory activity of CBD is the reduction of the concentraton of TNF-alpha in the synovium. It also reduces ROS that can increase inflammation and tissue damage. CBD also blocks nitric oxide production by the macrophages, which stimulates further inflammation. Through this process of immune modulation, CBD helps to inhibit inflammatory cell migration and infiltration into the tissue.[12, 13] Among the largest cells inhibited through migration and infiltration are the neutrophils.

CBD further reduces oxidative stress by reducing the production of ROS[12, 14] In this process, CBD helps reduce free radicals by blocking the activation of NADPH oxidase. CBD reduces the amount of TNF-alpha that is secreted and reduces the activation of p38MAPK. The result of these activities is a reduction in the spread and continuation of inflammation.

CBD has been shown to influence chondrocyte precursor cells. These mesenchymal stem cells[16] showed increased survival and migration to the site of tissue injury. CBD also led to chondrogenic differentiation from the mesenchymal stem cells. This process leads to the prevention of cartilage destruction.[11, 16-20]

Through his research, John McParland came to the conclusion that "the forces of embryogenesis become the forces of healing after birth."[21] He is referring here to the influence of the endocannabinoid system on fibroblasts. His work showed the extensive involvement of the endocannabinoid system in skeletal tissue repair.

Research shows that cannabinoid-based medicines[22] can help reduce pain with movement and pain at rest, as well as improve the quality of sleep. The pain reduction was from a suppression of the disease itself, along with a reduced perception of pain.

Cannabinoid receptor agonists reduce fibroblast-like synoviocytes (FLS) in both osteoarthritis and rheumatoid arthritis to reduce the production of IL-6 and IL-8[23], a proinflammatory cytokine and a proinflammatory chemokine, respectively. Reducing these is one avenue that some cannabinoids effect, thereby reducing the production of inflammatory cytokines. The reduction also helps reduce the propagation of inflammation and arthritis itself and can help prevent the destruction of cartilage.

Experiments showed that IL-6 and IL-8 were not blocked by CB1 or CB2 receptor agonists; therefore, this activity is independent of cannabinoid receptors. The cannabinoid agonists were independent of TRPV1 receptors and PPAR-gamma receptors and reduced IL-6 production in nonstimulated cells. The reduction was not shown for IL-8.

These are all of the receptors that have been documented to lead to the actions of cannabinoids. This information and these studies point to other methods of activity, perhaps through unknown cannabinoid receptors or mechanisms of which we are not presently aware.

IL-6[25] is the main driver of inflammation in rheumatoid arthritis. It induces osteoclast differentiation and leads to bone destruction and resorption. Endocannabinoids contribute to the regulation of bone mass.[26] This modulation of bone mass is important in arthritis because of the destruction of the bone under the cartilage. We might surmise that it's important as well when dealing with osteoporosis and osteopenia. Since cannabinoids help modulate bone density, this may provide another application for them.

The regulation of bone mass is felt to be modulated through the CB2 receptors present on both osteoblasts and osteoclasts. Research shows that CB2 receptor antagonism reduces osteoclastogenesis[24] and can be accomplished through the antagonism of both CB1 and CB2 receptors. With this activity, there is reduced formation and function of osteoclasts, the cells that break down bone. In the collagen-induced murine version of rheumatoid arthritis, the cannabinoids reduced the amount of inflammatory cytokines that were present. They also decreased antibody production, and, when begun early in the inflammatory process, they inhibited the formation of acute arthritis and reduced the amount of bone destruction.

The endocannabinoids are not limited to AEA and 2-AG. Other cannabinoids are seen in the tissues that do not react with cannabinoid CB1 or CB2 receptors and are referred to as "entourage" compounds.[27,28] Two of these compounds, OEA and PEA, are found in the joint but do not help modulate the endocannabinoid system through traditional receptors. PEA has anti-inflammatory activity through the PPAR-alpha receptors.[29] These receptors account for some of the entourage activity. They also help modulate nuclear transcription factors that help control metabolic processes and reduce inflammatory reactions. In a study looking at the tissues and synovial fluids of patients with osteoarthritis, rheumatoid arthritis, and normal joints, they were tested and compared. In both osteoarthritis and rheumatoid arthritis, AEA and 2-AG were found in the synovial fluid but not in normal synovial fluid. PEA was lower in osteoarthritis and rheumatoid arthritis than in normal joints.

The decrease in PEA may reflect the contribution of it to the disease process in osteoarthritis and rheumatoid arthritis. The progression of these diseases could be related to the loss of PEA through reduced production or degradation.

2-AG levels were lower in rheumatoid arthritis than in osteoarthritis in the synovial fluid. However, there was no difference in the levels found in the synovial tissue of the joints. Is there an imbalance in the production of cannabinoids that leads to the production and continuation of joint inflammation? Looking at the differences in the levels of endocannabinoids present in arthritic joints versus normal joints and the differences between rheumatoid arthritis and osteoarthritis, it seems plausible that variance in endocannabinoids presence reflects a problem.

Research shows that CB1 and CB2 receptors are coupled in some way to TRPV1,[30] and that linkage may be related to their activity. We are confident that the coupling is linked to the vasodilation effect in blood vessels in the knee joints. These are complicated interactions, though, not fully understood at this time. The issues with inflammation are further complicated by the regulation of cannabinoid receptor expression.[31,32] The receptor expression varies depending on the nature of the inflammatory stimulus and the tissue that is involved. When inflammation occurs, some tissues increase the number of cannabinoid receptors and other tissues reduce the number. Cannabinoid receptors appear to down-regulate in inflamed joints, which may be related to an up-regulation of stimulants, anandamide, 2-AG, or all three. Research shows that prolonged exposure to these compounds leads to some cannabinoid receptors being withdrawn back into the cells.[33, 34]

In summary, research indicates that the whole process of arthritis is linked to inflammation in complex ways. While the cause of these diseases is not completely known or understood at this time, research shows us that the cannabinoid compounds can be very helpful in reducing the inflammation, free radicals, nitric oxide, and immune-cell infiltration and activation. Given these outcomes, we believe further research and investigation into the application of these compounds is necessary and may result in CBD being one of the front-runners for the control of inflammation and pain that is related to arthritis.

XV

Cancer

Cancer is one of the most common diseases and killers today. Causes are numerous and may be biological, environmental, viral, or bacterial. There are also genetic predispositions to cancer; however, when you look at the broad majority of cancers, the cause is really unknown. This would include, among many others, breast, colon, rectum, lymph nodes, uterus, bladder, pancreas cancer, bone marrow, and stomach.[1]

Some of the most common and recognized environmental exposures that cause cancer are tobacco, polycyclic hydrocarbons, asbestos, arsenic, and vinyl chloride. These agents have been proven to be carcinogenic, and precautions have therefore been put into place for people who are exposed to them. Other physical agents that are carcinogens include ionizing radiation, ultraviolet radiation, and aflatoxin B1.

The next group of causes is viruses, many referred to as oncogenic because they can start and cause cancer. These viruses transform cells into a neoplastic state. This occurs when the cell is not a natural host. In a natural host, they are replicated and released. When the cell is nonpermissive (does not support the replication of a virus's mutant gene), the virus then takes control of the replicating process and the cell becomes neoplastic. The viral DNA can be inserted into cellular chromosomes; once inserted, the proteins for viral proliferation are produced.

Viruses have both early and late proteins, and the viral genes also help maintain the transformation. The retroviruses are the most well-known of these oncogenic ribonucleic acid (RNA) viruses. They carry their own reverse transcriptase so they can convert their RNA into deoxyribonucleic acid (DNA), which can then be incorporated into the cellular DNA and be replicated. These viruses carry three genes: group-specific antigens, internal structural proteins, and envelope proteins.

One of the subtypes of these RNA retroviruses is the human T-cell leukemia virus (HTLV), either type I or type II. Another virus in this category is the human immunodeficiency virus (HIV), also referred to as lentivirus. Infection with this virus also predisposes the individual to other opportunistic infections.

Oncogenic DNA viruses include papovavirus, simian virus 40, adenoviruses, herpes viruses, Epstein-Barr virus, hepatitis B virus, hepatitis C virus, human papilloma virus (HPV) type 16 and 18, and human herpes virus-8 (HHV 8) (also known as also known as Kaposi sarcoma-associated herpes virus, or KSHV). These viruses have DNA, and they can they can directly insert it into our cellular DNA.

Bacterial causes of cancer include the *Helicobacter pylori*. This bacterium can cause gastritis and lead to ulcers and cancer formation. Other bacteria can cause cancer, but they have not been as well studied as *H. pylori*.

In our normal cellular DNA, we have the precursors for cancer development. We have oncogenes and proto-oncogenes, both of which can be activated through replication. These are matching homolog's two retroviral oncogenes. There are no introns, the segments that begin replication in retroviral oncogenes; these segments get changes from proto-oncogenes if and when they become associated. Proto-oncogenes produce very specific compounds that can be growth factors, growth factor receptors, or signal transducer proteins and are known to function in normal cells. We also have tumor suppressor genes that control autophagy and apoptosis.[1] Produced modulators of the cell cycle called cycline proteins help modulate the speed of cell cycles. Cycline-dependent kinases are compounds that stop the cell cycle between G1, the resting phase, and S phase, which is for DNA synthesis.

Some human cancers are known to be derived from proto-oncogene. These include Burkitt's lymphoma, chronic myeloid leukemia, bladder carcinoma, some lung and colon carcinomas, and neuroblastoma. These have all been shown to be derived from the activation of normal proto-oncogenes.[1] In some cases cellular proto-oncogenes convert to oncogenes. When this occurs their activation forms cancers. They can be produced from genetic translocation, promoter insertion, point mutations of the DNA, and delusional mutations and amplification.[1]

We all carry the potential to develop cancers in our DNA. When our immune system is functioning normally, these cancers are immediately destroyed. However, when the immune system is not functionally normally, these cancers can escape detection and destruction.

Epigenetics is the study of cellular changes that occur but are not related to changes in the DNA and is another area that addresses the occurrence of cancer.[2] Epigenetics describes cellular potential for change and a response to changes in the environment that can modulate DNA translation and reflects the cells' unlimited potential. Every cell in our body has the same DNA, but the expression of that DNA is unique to each cell, tissue, and organ. It is the epogenome that aids in turning off and on of particular genes in particular tissues. For example, the DNA in our hair, eyes, and fingernails are all the same except that different genes are turned on and off, giving them individual characteristics. Part of the epigenome activity is through biochemical modification that include methylation and the histone wrapping of DNA.

These two categories of modifications turn genes on and off. This whole process changes with age, and the number of times a cell has divided will affect its susceptibility to cancer. The more cells divide, the more likely we are to develop inflammation and have reduced stem-cell vitality and ability to repair damage.[2]

Cancer is very prevalent throughout the world, with the highest prevalence in North America, where it is estimated that 1.5 percent of the population greater than 15 years old has or will have cancer. That calculates to about 3.2 million individuals affected. In Western Europe 1.2 percent of their population 15 years of age and older, or 3.9 million individuals, is affected, and in Japan it's 1 percent of their population.

The basic treatments for cancer include surgery, radiation therapy, and chemotherapy, and then follow-up that is determined by the type of cancer that is treated. Our basic treatments of cancer are not very successful; side effects from radiation therapy and chemotherapy are devastating by themselves. Cancer treatment is often a process of trying to kill the cancer before you kill the person.

Cannabinoids and their potency as anticancer agents has been researched mainly outside of the United States. The reason for that is current US government's policy on marijuana and the government's need to show that there is no medical benefit to marijuana. For this reason, only certain types of cancers have been studied and many others not.[32] Cannabinoids are potent anticancer agents because they modulate many of the key signaling pathways, including growth, differentiation, angiogenesis (the growth of new blood vessels), and metastasis.

Some tumors are very susceptible to cannabinoid-induced growth inhibition.[4,32,33] These include lung carcinoma, glioma, thyroid epithelioma, lymphoma, leukemia, skin carcinoma, uterine carcinoma, breast carcinoma, prostate carcinoma, neuroblastoma, colorectal cancer. Through the manipulation of growth and its inhibition, cannabinoids can reduce tumor bulk and metastatic disease.

Cannabinoid activity with possible antitumor functions includes modulation of adenylyl cyclase activity in the modulation of intracellular c-AMP. Another factor that can contribute to antitumor activity is the modulation of protein kinase A (PKA) a protein kinase pathway. This pathway modulates Ca2+ and K+ channels and can modulate neurotransmitter release. Other pathways also can affect cell fate. These include stimulation of the MAPK pathway, extracellular-signal-regulated kinase (ERK), which is similar to and functions with the MAPK pathway, and then stress-activated kinases. The stress-activated kinases can contribute to cell growth, differentiation, autophagy, and apoptosis. They can also affect the phosphoinositide 3-kinase (PI3K)-Akt survival pathway. Control of this pathway can contribute to cell survival or cell death. Stress-activated kinases can also stimulate ceramide production de novo, meaning the natural cellular production, not by outside stimulation. This ceramide production can activate other stress proteins and lead to the loss of mitochondrial function.

The cannabinoids have been shown to induce apoptosis of tumor cells while protecting normal cells from any damage. Cannabinoids inhibit the growth of transformed cells and prevent the tumors from angiogenesis. They also are capable of inhibiting the metastasis of cancers and growth factor receptor signaling.

In endothelial cells, which are the cells that produce blood vessels, cannabinoids control their size, their ability to differentiate, and their permeability. Cannabinoids prevent endothelial cell migration and cancer cell migration,[33, 40] inhibit cell adhesion, prevent invasion of surrounding tissues, and inhibit the cancer's ability to metastasize. Cannabinoids also decrease the life of the endothelial cells, making them mature quickly and become impermeable.

Much of the activity that the cannabinoids carry out is through a known group of receptors.[34, 35] These include cannabinoid receptors CB1 and CB2, TRPV1,[36] putative cannabinoid receptors, the orphan G-protein coupled receptor 55 (GPR55),[37] and the PPAR-gamma and 5HT1A receptors.[33] In worldwide research, these are the most common receptors that have been shown to interact with cannabinoids, but many actions that are seen with these compounds must be carried out by other receptors or other methods that we are not aware of presently.

The effects of these compounds vary with the type of cancer cells with which they interact. Each cell type has its own susceptibility or resistance to the cannabinoids. Different receptors are used in different cell types, and in some tissues the activities are independent of receptors. CBD is the most potent cannabinoid used against cancers. It has no psychotropic effects and has a very low toxic profile. We will now look at some of the cancer types that respond well and see the mechanism of action and exactly what happens in most cell types.

Gliomas are one of the most difficult cancers to treat.[4] Even with the best radiological, surgical, and chemo therapies, the median survival is less than one year.[11] The first report of the use of delta-9-THC was reported in 1998. It was shown that THC was very active against gliomas,[12] and that this was not mediated by CB1 receptors.[33] There was partial CB2 receptor activity that decreased proliferation of the glioma cells. It was further shown that this activity was not carried out through TRPV1 receptors, but that the THC generated ROS in the tumor cells, which led to their death.[33] An elevation in ceramide production was also noted. There were two peaks of elevation—one happening within minutes with a two-fold increase in ceramide, and the other seen days after the treatment with a four-fold increase. It was later learned that the ceramide elevation in the second peak was due to de novo synthesis of ceramide, which increased the production of stress-regulated protein p8. The elevation of p8 leads to the activation of proapoptotic pathways.[13–16] In addition, the injection of cannabinoids into the gliomas prolonged the individual survival and completely eradicated tumor in 20 to 35 percent of the treated animals in studies.[13]

Further studies of gliomas showed that the cannabinoids exerted control over cell proliferation and survival pathways. In controlling the ERK-1 and ERK-2 pathways, they decreased proliferation, cell migration, and invasiveness.[5,33] They also exerted control over the PI3K/Akt pathway,[8,33] which can also decrease proliferation, reduce migration, and eliminate invasion. CBD was shown to decrease the activity of 5-lipoxygenase and thus decrease proliferation, migration, and invasion.

CBD was also shown to decrease the amount of FAAH, which is the enzyme that degrades our common endocannabinoids. With this action, there is an increase in anandamide, which stimulates the CB1 receptors. The combination of CBD and anandamide decrease the proliferation, migration, and invasion by cancer cells. It increases the production of ROS in tumor cells, as well as decreases cellular glutathione, which makes the tumor cells more sensitive to oxidative stress, and triggers apoptosis or autophagy.

Cannabinoids affect the focal adhesion kinases[9] that affect a cancer's ability to grow and spread. Inability to grow and spread will stimulate an increase in oxidative stress and the production of free radicals. The free-radical increase will lead to an increase in activation of caspase-9 and -8. The activation of these two compounds increased and activated caspase-3, leading to mitochondrial dysfunction. This mitochondrial dysfunction will in turn lead to a leaking of the cytochrome c into the cytoplasm from the mitochondria, with an additional reduction in the membrane potential of the mitochondria, leading to a collapse in energy production.

These compounds decrease the production of hypoxia-inducible transcription factor 1 alpha (HIF-1alpha).[33,45] With the decrease in this compound, a cell has difficulty in responding to hypoxia and oxidative stress, which contributes to a decrease in proliferation, migration, and invasion. In these studies, it was shown that cannabinoids selectively affect tumor cells and do not affect normal brain cells.[17,18] They actually have been shown to protect normal neurons. In some studies, the stimulation of CB2 cannabinoid receptors were shown to induce tumor regression.[19]

In many studies CBD was chosen over THC because of its nonpsychotropic effects, and in some of the earliest ones, CBD was shown to inhibit human glioma cells.[20] This ambition was dose-dependent, led to apoptosis, and was accomplished through the induction of overwhelming oxidative stress.[18,37,41-44] These studies also showed that CBD led to depletion of glutathione from the tumor cells. This induction of ROS-stimulated apoptosis could be reversed through the antioxidant tocopherol.[37] All the activities of CBD were independent of the known receptors.[20]

CBD was shown to increase the release of cytochrome c from the mitochondria into the cell cytoplasm. The activation of caspases-8, -9 and -3 led to the activation of both the intrinsic and extrinsic apoptotic pathways. In essence, this happens because of CBD's ability to disrupt mitochondrial function, leading to the activation of the intrinsic pathway and disruption of nuclear and other cell functions to activate the extrinsic pathway. This is further assisted with the down-regulation of signaling molecules for tumor cell proliferation.[33, 45] These proliferation pathways include ERK and PI3K/Akt. With the blocking of these pathways, the cells' ability to respond to stress and proliferate is reduced. The hypoxia-inducible transcription factor is blocked as well, which reduces the cells' ability to respond to the hypoxia and increase free radicals. A couple of studies showed that combinations of CBD with THC causes cellular death at lower doses than either one was capable of causing by itself. This was accomplished through cell-cycle arrest and increased production of ROS. The cell death was accomplished through the sustained activation of caspases -3, -7, and -9, which assist in the breakdown of mitochondrial function.

THC was shown to increase intracellular accumulation of ceramide through de novo synthesis. This process leads to apoptosis, and ceramide levels are inversely correlated with malignant progression in glial tumors and poor prognosis.[21] With increased levels of ceramide, there is increased expression of the P8 transcription factor, thus inducing endoplasmic reticulum stress and the production of activating transcription factor 4 (ATF4) and cyclophosphamide, doxorubicin, Oncovin (vincristine), and prednisone (CHOP). These two stress compounds increase the activation of pseudokinase tribbles homolog 3 (TRB3). This compound converges on the mitochondria to trigger the intrinsic pathway to apoptosis. This is combined with the activation of the caspases.[16]

Multiple cannabinoids acting through CB1 receptors can down-regulate pathways and growth factors that reduce tumor cells' ability to survive.[22] These pathways are activated by some cannabinoids independent of receptor activity. In their endeavor to grow and expand, all cancer cells must have new blood-vessel growth and migration ability.[4] At first they must grow locally, then spread locally with the potential for metastasis to distant sites. Angiogenesis is required for this whole process to occur, and angiogenesis requires the proliferation and migration of endothelial cells, the ability to manipulate the extracellular matrix, then the morphologic differentiation of the endothelial cells to form tubes. Multiple factors are required in the proper timing and sequence for this to occur.

Cannabinoids inhibit angiogenesis, which also enables them to metastasize.[22,23] These compounds change the blood-vessel morphology and control pathways that modulate the activity of new vessel formation. They reduce the production of vascular endothelial growth factor (VEGF), and the production and activation of the VEGF receptor. In doing so, cannabinoids can then control the formation and activity of new blood vessels. They further inhibit the migration of vascular endothelial cells.[24] This activity inhibits cell migration of the endothelial cells and reduces their survival. Success in accomplishing this depends on the CBD dose: lower doses stop migration while a larger dose is necessary to produce apoptosis.[25] CBD's activity helps to further regulate the expansion through other tissues.

CBD down-regulates the expression of tissue inhibitors of metalloproteinases (TIMPs).[26, 27] The metalloproteinases are compounds that enable cells to break down the intercellular matrix and are needed for both expansion of the tumor cells and the invasion of blood vessels. Through this control of TIMPs, CBD controls tumor growth, angiogenesis, and metastasis. Tumors cannot expand if they cannot degrade the extracellular matrix.

CBD causes the release of apoptotic enzymes and the cleavage of cell surface receptors. It decreases tumor-cell proliferation, migration, adhesion, and dispersion, which in turn prevents the tumor from growing and spreading beyond the limits when CBD is started. By preventing new blood-vessel formation and increasing the host defense mechanisms, CBD further enhances the destruction of the tumor. With the inhibition of angiogenesis this is accomplished through the inhibition of endothelial cell migration and survival, when you cannot produce functional endothelial cells for blood vessels then there is no cell migration or survival.[28-31]

The cannabinoids alter gene expression. They protect the development of glioma-derived stem-like cells. By supporting and controlling these cells, cannabinoids help to create proliferation of glioma cells and to modulate their differentiation into the forms that are needed. They reduce glioma tumor-cell proliferation, one of the cancers that is suspected to be stem cells.[4] The tumors suspected of derived from stem-cell duration include gliomas, and hematopoietic, breast, and prostate tumors.

Breast Cancer

In 2006 Ligresti et al. showed that CBD potently and selectively inhibited breast-cancer cell growth[48] and reduced infiltration of lung metastasis. Their work showed that this was accomplished through TRPV1 receptors and CB2 receptors through indirect activation by way of FAAH.[49] They also showed the induction of oxidative stress. Through the activity modulated through the receptors, CBD blocked cell proliferation, invasion, and metastasis.

Of the cannabinoids tested, CBD was the most effective at suppressing breast cancer, and it was shown to down-regulate the ID-1 gene.[49] The ID-1 gene is what controls the invasiveness of breast cancer and its ability to metastasize. By blocking this gene, CBD prevents proliferation of breast cancer, and the migration and invasion in surrounding tissues. CBD was also shown to mediate up-regulation of extracellular signal-regulated ERK.[33, 42] This control led to increased ROS and further reduced cell proliferation. CBD also reduced primary tumor mass and the number of metastatic foci.

Tests demonstrated that CBD was active against both estrogen-positive and estrogen-negative breast cancer.[33, 43] The activity of CBD was independent of CB1, CB2, and TRPV receptor activation and did not affect normal nontumor cells. The CBD induced both autophagy, which is the recycling of normal cell constituents, and apoptosis. The activities of autophagy and apoptosis remediated through increased endoplasmic retriculum stress from inhibiting Akt/mTOR/4EBP1 signaling.

This increases ROS, which in turn reduces the cells' ability to compensate for these compounds. A reduction in mitochondrial membrane potential then leads to the reduction of energy production for the cancer cells.

The mitochondrial decline is marked by the translocation of Beclin-2 and its interaction with mitochondrial proteins, and the introduction of Bid into the mitochondria itself. There is leakage through the mitochondrial membranes, and holes are punched that allow the release of cytochrome c into the cytoplasm. This activity activates the apoptotic pathway, also known as the suicide pathway. If you inhibit the activation of the caspases, this would lead to reduced apoptosis. However, with this reduction there was a rebalancing and an increase in autophagy. This modulation was carried out by Beclin-1. CBD increases the cleavage of Beclin-1.[50, 51] Through this cleavage, there was an increase in the cleavage of Bid and this was translocated into the mitochondria. The movement of Bid into the mitochondria creates further leakage of cytochrome c from the mitochondria into the cell cytoplasm. This loss of cytochrome c leads to a failure in the production of energy in the cancer cells, and they can no longer survive.

The Beclin-1 cleavage leads to fragments being translocated into the mitochondria.[33,43,50,51] These fragments lead to cytochrome c leakage and trigger apoptosis. The combination of these processes leads to a decrease in cancer-cell proliferation and all activity that would support cell life. In this stress state and with the genes turned off, there can be no invasion or metastasis.

Leukemia and Lymphoma

Leukemia and lymphoma are immune-system tumors, and the immune system is heavily favored with CB2 receptors,[53] making these tumors some of the most responsive to cannabinoids. In early studies CBD was shown to induce apoptosis by the activation of caspase-3 through a CB2 receptor activation[33,52] CBD also caused activation of caspase-8 and -9 in response to its ability to create free radicals in the cancer cells, leading to apoptosis and reduced proliferation. The Bid present in the cells was fragmented, and some of those fragments were transported into the mitochondria, which led to reduced mitochondrial membrane potential. With this there was no longer an efficient electron transport, leading to a reduction in energy production and an increase in free-radical generation. This was also accompanied by leakage of the cytochrome c from the mitochondria into the cytoplasm. With this release of cytochrome c from the mitochondria leading to a breakdown in mitochondrial function, more ROS was created. CBD also reduces levels of p38MAPK,[52] which leads to a reduction in cell differentiation and further apoptosis.

Studies demonstrated that immune cells were much more sensitive to CBD than to THC. For THC to be effective, a concentration of 10 micromoles or greater is needed to induce apoptosis in immune cells. This was accomplished by the activation of caspase-2, -8, -9, and -10. Through this activation, the intrinsic pathway was activated from mitochondrial damage. In the cytoplasm, Bid cleaved, with fragments being transported in the mitochondria, leading to the leakage of cytochrome c into the cytoplasm.

THC also led to an increase in ceramide. This increase led to a loss of mitochondrial membrane potential, which created a loss of cellular energy and the leakage of cytochrome c into the cytoplasm. It also produced phosphorylation of Raf-1, mitogen-activated protein kinase-1 (MEK-1) and -2 and ERK-1 and -2. The phosphorylation of these compounds leads to an increase in the development of apoptosis.

The combination of these activities leads to the decrease in proliferation and invasion of the immune-based cancers. Due to the high receptor concentrations for cannabinoids, the response to CBD was quick, and, in the studies, low concentrations of CBD were very effective.

Lung cancer

Studies of lung cancer showed that CBD reduces the invasiveness of the cancers.[54-56] The activity included CB1, CB2, and TRPV1 receptors and an up-regulation of tissue inhibitor of MMP-1. The up-regulation of TIMP1 led to decreased invasiveness and decreased angiogenesis. With this in place, it was difficult for the lung cancers to inlarge and to metastasize.

The increase in TIMP1 was induced by a couple of mechanisms. The induction of p38MAPK and an increase in ERK both led to an increase in the amount of TIMP1 that was produced and greatly limited lung cancer's ability to change the matrix and send out new blood vessels to increase its size. Also shown was a reduction of plasminogen activator inhibitor-1 (PAI-1). This compound is critical to invasion by the cancer cells. Blocking PAI-1 reduced the cells' ability to spread and take over more tissue.[55]

CBD at concentrations as low as 0.01 to 0.05 micromoles/ liter, 1×10^{-6} was able to decrease metastasis up to 84 percent. This study showed both the effectiveness of CBD and the low doses at which it can be used for treatment.

Colon Cancer

The study of colon cancer has been done in animals and is induced by the compound azoxymethane (AOM).[57] This compound induces aberrant cryptic foci and polyps, followed by tumor formation. This model exactly reflects human colon cancer. Cannabinoids induced up-regulation of phosphor-Akt, iNOS, and COX-2. This regulation system starts the modified ROS production. It prevents free radicals, thereby reducing the formation of precursors to colon cancer. There was a down-regulation of caspase-3.[56-58]

Studies with CBD at the dosage of 1 mg/kg showed reduced aberrant cryptic foci formation. At a dose of 5 mg/kg, polyps and tumors were reduced. In this animal model, CBD was shown to be capable of both the treatment of the cancer and prevention of the formation of cancer.[57–58]

The dose of 1 mg/kg reversed the protective effects of phosphor-Akt. It also reversed the activity and protection of caspase-3, which led to an increase in free radicals in the mitochondria and the destruction of the mitochondria itself, leaving the tumor cells without energy.[58]

A comparative study between CBD and delta-9-THC showed that, used in in combination, they had a greater effect at a lower dose. It was shown that this combination helped reduce iNOS but did not affect COX-2.[57]

2-AG, which provides stimulation of CB1 receptors, also increased. This stimulation helps provide more antiproliferative effects. Anandamide, which acts at both CB1 and TRPV1 receptors, increased as well. Part of this increase was due to the blocking of the enzyme FAAH, which breaks down anandamide and some 2-AG.[58]

It was shown that CBD protected normal cells and the cells' DNA from oxidative damage. There was no genotoxic damage from the CBD, and CBD reduced intestinal contractility. The other effect of CBD is reduction of intestinal inflammation.[57, 58]

Studies show that it is the combination of CBD and THC that is the most effective in treating colon cancer. Most of the research that has been done has been carried on outside of the United States because of the status of marijuana in the United States. There are now companies that are producing synthetic cannabinoids, which are being studied and used under the funding of the drug companies.

Our knowledge of this whole endocannabinoids system must include the understanding that it is the balance in cell activity that is required for health, and too much or too little leads to dysfunction of the systems. The activity of the cells affected by this imbalance will depend on the cell type. The receptors found in the cells will influence their responsiveness or resistance to cannabinoid treatment.

It has been my goal to highlight some of the research that has been done and demonstrate that this research shows that marijuana does have medicinal effects. Closing our eyes to this leads only to the ill health of our population. It is my hope that science and true scientific discovery will override the prejudices that exist at this present moment. There is much that can be done and will be done in the future. My only hope is that we are participants in this discovery process, which is actually only the rediscovery of a true gift that has been given us for our health.

Summary

I hope this book has provided you with some insight and information into the benefits of medicinal cannabis. Based on only a fraction of the research that has been completed, we have outlined the various benefits and described their method of action for some diseases. Cannabinoids act through many mechanisms using many different receptors. Their activity is both central and peripheral, each cannabinoid having its specific range of benefits.

It is time to remove our blinders, release our prejudices, and focus on the benefits that are offered for so many diseases. It will be through further research that we will tease out the actual pathways and benefits for each cannabinoid. Eventually, it will be the combinations of multiple cannabinoids that will give us the greatest benefits.

References

HISTORY OF HEMP

1. "10,000-year History of Marijuana use in the World," Advanced Holistic Health, accessed August 29, 2015, http://www.advancedholistichealth.org/history.html.

2. "Hemp's History," Truth About Hemp, accessed August 29, 2015, http://www.truthabouthemp.org/history.html.

3. "The History of Hemp," Hemp History, accessed August 29, 2015, http://www.globalhemp.com/2001/01/hemp-history.html.

4. "Hemp Since the Beginning of Time," Global Hemp, accessed August 29, 2015, http://www.globalhemp.com/2001/01/hemp-history.html.

5. Sagan, Carl. "Dragons of Eden Speculations on the Evolution of Human Intelligence" (Random House Publishing, 2012) p191 footnote.

6. Head, Tom, "Marijuana Laws in the United States," Civil Liberty, accessed August 29, 2015, http://civilliberty.about.com/od/drugpolicy/tp/Marijuana-History-Laws-United-States.htm.

7. "The Truth About Marijuana," The Vaults of Erowid, accessed August 29, 2015, http://erowid.org/plants/cannabis_culture11.shtml.

8. "Nabilone," Drugs, accessed August 29, 2015, http://drugs.com/mtm/nabilone.html.

9. Judge Young, Francis L., "Marijuana Rescheduling Petition," Docket No. 86–22, http://ccguide.org/young88.php.

10. "Official U.S. Report Backs Medical Use of Marijuana", National Academy of Sciences Institute of Medical Report on Medical Cannabis, March 17, 1999, http://www.levellers.org/iompr.htm.

INFLAMMATION

1. Janeway, C., Travers, P., Walport, M., Capra, J. Immuniobiology: The Immune System in Health and Disease. 6th Edition. New York, N.Y: Garland Publishers. 2005.

2. McGuirk, P., Mills, K.H.G. Pathogen specific regulatory T cells provoke a shift in the Th1/Th2 paradigm in immunity to infectious diseases. Trends in Immunology. 2002; 23(9): 450–55.

3. Stix,G. Is chronic inflammation the key to unlocking the mysteries of cancer? Scientific American November 9,2008.

4. J.F.Foley, Focus Issue: Understanding Mechanisms of Inflammation. Sci. Signal. 6, eg2(2013).

5. Tang, D., Kang, R., Coyne, C.B., Zeh, H.J., Lotze, M.T. PAMPs and DAMPs: signal 0s that spur autophagy and immunity. Immunol. Rev. 2012; 249(1): 158–75. Doi:10.1111/j.1600–065X.2012.01146.x.

6. Theoides, T.C., Alysendrates, K.D., Ansalidou, A., Delivanis, D.A., Sisunopoulous, N., Zhang, B., et al. Mast cells and inflammation. Biochem. Biophys. ACTA. 2012; 1822(1): 21–33. doi: 10.1016/j.bbadio2010.12014.

7. Cawthorn, W.P., Sethi, P. TNF-alpha and adipocyte biology. FEBS Lett. 2008; 582(1): 117–31.

8. Perera, M.K., Herath, N.P., Pathirana, S.L., Phone-Kyaw, M., Alles, H.K., et al. Association of high plasma TNF-alpha levels and TNF-alpha/IL-10 ratios with TNF2 allele in severe P. falciparum malaria patients in Sri Lanka. Pathogens and Global Health. 2013; 107(1): 21–29.

9. Feldman, A.M., Combes, A., Wagner, D., Kadakomi, T., Kubota, T., et al. The role of tumor necrosis factor in the pathophysiology of heart failure. J.. Am. Col.Cardiology. 2000; 35(3): 537–44. Doi: 10.1016/S0735-1097(99)00600-2.

10. Esposito, E., Cuzzocrea, S. TNF-alpha as a therapeutic target in inflammatory disease, ischemia-reperfusion injury and trauma. Curr. Med. Chem. 2009; 16(24): 3152–67.

11. http://www.bio.davidson.edu/courses/immuniology/students/spring2000/wolf/tnfalpha.html.

12. Payne, V., Kam, P.C. Mast cell tryptase: a review of its physiology and clinical significance. Anesthesia 2004; 59(7): 695–703.

13. Hancock, J.T., Desikan, D., Neill, S.J. Role of Reactive Oxygen species in cell signaling pathways. Biochemical and Biomedical aspects of Oxidative Modification 2001; 29(2): 345–50.

14. Burhans, W., Heintz, N. The cell cycle is a redox cycle: Linking phase specific targets to cell fate. Free Radical Biol. and Med. 2009; 47:1282–94.

15. Maintz, L., Novak, N. Histamine and histamine intolerance 1'2'3. Am. J. Clin. Nutrition. 2007; 85(5): 1185–96.

16. Dinarello, C.A. Immunological and inflammatory functions of the interleukin-1 family. Annu. Rev. Immunol. 2009; 27: 519–50. Doi: 10.1146/annurev.immunol.021908.132612.

17. Golias, Ch., Charalabopoulos, A.,Stagikas, D., Charalabopoulous, K., Batistatou, A. The kinin system-bradykinin: biological effects and clinical implications. Multiple role of the kinin system. Hippokratia. 2007; 11(3): 124–28.

18. Agostoni, A., Cugno, M. The kinin system: biological medcchanisms and clinical implications. Recent Prog. Med. 2001; 92: 764–73.

19. Funk, C.D. Prostaglandins and leukotrienes: advances in Eicosanoid biology. Science. 2001; 294(5548): 1871–75. Doi:10.1126/science.294.5548.1871.

20. Stedman's Medical Dictionary (twenty-seventh ed.) Williams and Wilkins. 2000.

21. Rather, L.J. Disturbance of function (function laesa): the fifth cardinal sign of inflammation, added by Galen to the four cardinal signs of Celsus. Bull N Y Acad. Med. 1971; 47(3): 303–22.https; //www.ncbi.nlm.nih.gov/pmc/articles/PMC1749862.

22. Cotran; Kumar,Collins (1998). Robbins Pathologic Basis of Disease. Philadelphia: W.B .Saunders Company. ISBN 0–7216-7335-X.33 http://bme.virginia.edu/key/main.html.

23. Eming, S.A., Krieg, T., Davidson, J.M. Inflammation in wound repair: molecular and cellular mechanisms. J. Investig. Dermatol. 2007; 127 (3): 5134–25. Doi:10.1038/sj.jid.5700701.

24. Ashcroft, G.S., Yang, X., Glick, A.B., Weinstein, M., Letterio, J.J., Mizel, D.E., et al. Mice lacking Smad3 show accelerated wound healing and an impaired local inflammatory response. Nat. Cell Biol. 1999; 1(5): 260–66. Doi: 10.1038/1297.

25. Ashcroft, G.S. Bidirectional regulation of macrophage function by TGF-Beta. Microbes Infect. 1999; 1(15): 1275–82. Doi: 10.1016/S1286-4579(99)00257-9.

26. Werner, F., Jain, M.K., Feinberg, M.W., Sibinga, N.E., Pellacani, A., et al. Transforming growth factor-Beta 1 inhibition of macrophage activation is mediated via Smad3. J. Biol. Chem. 2000; 275(47): 36653–58.

27. Sato, Y., Ohshima,T., Kondo, T. Regulatory role of endogenous interleukin-10 in cutaneous inflammatory response of murine wound healing. Biochem. Biophys. Res. Commun. 1999; 265(1): 194–99. Doi: 10.1006.anbbrc.1999.1455.

28. Serhan, C.N. Controlling the solution of aute inflammation: a new genus of dual anti-inflammatory and proresolving mediators. J. PERIODONTAL. 2008; 79(8Suppl)): 1520–26. Doi: 10.1902/jop.2008.080231.

29. Greenhalgh, D.G. The role of apoptosis in wound healing. Int. J. Biochem. Cell Biol. 1998; 30(9): 1019–30.

30. Jiang, D., Liang, J., Fan, J., Yu,S., Chen, S., Luo, Y., et al. Regulation of lung injury and repair by Toll-like receptors and hyaluronan. Nat. Med. 2005; 11(11): 1173–79.

31. Teder, P., Vandiver, R.W., Jiang, D., Liang, J., Cohn, L., Pure, E., et al. Resolution of lung inflammation by CD44. Science. 2002; 296(5565): 155–58.

32. McCawley, L.J., Matrisin, L.M. Matrix metalloproteinases: they're not just for the matrix anymore! Curr. Opin. Cell Biol. 2001; 13: 534–40.

33. Seaman, D.R. The diet-induced proinflammatory state: a cause of chronic pain and other degenerative diseases? J. Manipulative Physiol. Ther. 2002; 25(3): 168–79.

ENDOCANNABINOID SYSTEM

1. Sulak, D. Introduction to the Endocannabinoid system. http://normal.org/library/item/introduction-to-the-endocannabinoid-system.

2. Mechoula, R., Shvo,Y. The structure of cannabadiol. Tetrahedron 1963; 19: 2073–78.

3. Gaoni, Y., Mechoulam, R. Isolation, structure, and partial synthesis of an active constituient of hashish. J. Am. Chem. Soc., 1964; 86: 1946.

4. Griffing, G.T. Endocannabinoids Overview. http://emedicine.medscape.com/article/1361971-overview#a1.

5. Matsuda, L.A., Lolait, SJ, Brownstein, MJ, Young, AC, Bonner, TI. Strtucture of a cannabinoid receptor and functional expression of the cloned cDNA. Nature; 1990; 346:561–4.

6. Devane, WA., Hanus, L., Breuer, A., Pertwee, RG., Stevenson, LA.,Griffin, G., etal. Isolation and structure of a brain constituent that binds to the cannabinoid receptor. Science. Dec 18 1992; 258(5090):1946–9.

7. Munro, S, Thomas, AL, Abu Shaar, M. Molecular characterization of a peripheral receptor for cannabinoids. Nature 1993; 365:61–5.

8. Sugiura, T, Kondo, S, Sukagawa, A, Shinoda,A, Itoh, K, et al. 2_Arachidonoylglyerol: a possible endogenous cannabinoid receptor ligand in brain. Biochem Biophys Res Commun 1995; 215:89–97.

9. Mechoulam,R, Ben Shabat, S, Hanus, L, Ligumsky, M, Kaminski, NE, SCHATZ, AR, et al. Isolation of an endogenous 2-monoglyceride, present in canine gut, that binds to cannabinoid receptors. Biochem Pharmacol 1995; 50:83–90.

10. Onaivi, ES, Ishiguro, H, Liu, Q-R, Gong, J-P, Tagliaferro,P, Brusco, A, Arinami,T, Uhl, GR, CNS Effects of CB2 Cannabinoid Receptors. The Open Neuropsychopharmacology J. 2009; 2:45–52.

11. Goldman, N. "An overview of the endogenous Cannabinoid System: Components and Possible Roles of this Recently Discovered Regulatory System". Erowid.org, v1.1 May 2003,v1.2 Feb 2005. http://www.erowid.org/plants/cannabis/cannabis_pharmacology2.shtml.

12. Turu, G., Hunyady, L. Signal transduction of the CB1 cannabinoid receptor. J Molecular Endocrinology.2010; 44:75–85. Doi:10.1677/jme-08–0190.

13. Svizenska, I., Dubovy, P., Sulcova, A. Cannabinoid receptors 1 and 2 (CB1 and CB2), their distribution, ligands and functional involvement in nervous system structures—A short review. Pharm Biochem and Behavior. 2008; 90:501–11.

14. Mackie,K. Distribution of Cannabinoid receptors in the Central and Peripheral Nervous System. HEP 2005; 168:299–325.

15. Glass, M, Dragunow, M, Faull, RL, Cannabinoid reeptors in the human brain: a detailed anatominical and quantative autoradiograph study in the fetal, neonatal and adult human brain. Neuroscience 1997; 77:299–318.

16. Mato, S, Del Olmo, E, Pazos, A., Ontogenetic development of the cannabinoid receptor expression and signal transduction functionality in the human brain. Eur J Neurosci. 2003; 17: 1747–1754.

17. Cabral, GA, Marijuana and Cannabinoids: Effects on Infections, Immunity, and AIDS. Cannabis Therapeutics in HIV/AIDS, 2001 the Hawthorne Press.

18. Duncan,M, Mouihate, A, Mackie, K., Keenan, CM, Buckley, NE, Davison,JS, Patel, KD, Pittman, QJ, Sharkey, KA. Cannabinoid CB2 receptors in the enteric nervous system modulate gastrointestinal motility in Lipopolysaccharide-treated rats. Am J Physiol Gastrointest Liver Physiol2008; 295: G78-G87. Doi:10.1152/ajpgi.90285.2008.

19. Smith, PB, Compton, DR, Welch, SP, Razdan, RK, Martin, BR, The pharmacological activity of anandamide, a putative endogenous cannabinoid, in mice. J Pharmacol Exp Ther. 1994; 270:219–27.

20. Romero,J, Garcia, L, Fernandez-Ruis, JJ, Cebeira, M, Ramos, JA, Changes in rat brain cannabinoid binding sites after acute or chronic exposure to their endogenous agonist, anandamide, or to delta-9-tetrahydrocannabinol. Pharm Biochem Behav. 1995; 51:731–7.

21. Mechoulam, R, Ben-Shabat, S, Hanus, L, Ligumsky, M, Schatz, AK, Gopher, A, Almog, S, Martin, BR, Compton, DR, Pertwee, RG, Griffin, G, Bayewitch, M, Barg,J, Vogel, Z. Identification of an endogenous 2-monoglyceride, present in canine gut, that binds to cannabinoid receptors. Biochem Pharmacol. 1995; 50:83–90.

22. Lee, M, Yang, KH, Kaminski, NE, Effects of putative cannabinoid receptor ligands, anandamide and 2-arachidonoyl-glycerol on immune function in B6C3F1 splenocytes. J Pharmacol Exp Ther. 1995; 275:529–536.

23. Facci,L, Dal Toso, R, Romanello, S, Buriani,A, Skaper, SD, Leon, A, Mast cells express a peripheral cannabinoid receptor with differential sensitivity to anandamide and palmitoylethanolamide. Proc Natl Acad Sci USA. 1995; 92:3376–3380.

24. Hanus, L., Gopher,A., Almog, S., Mechoulam R. Two new unsaturated fatty acid ethanolamides in brain that bind to the cannabinoid receptor. J Med Chem. 1993; 36:3032–3034.

25. Rinaldi-Carmoni, M, Barth,F, Heaulme, M, shire,D, calandra, B, Congy, C, Martinez,S, Maurani,J, Neliat, G, Ferrara, P, Soubrie, P, Brelier, JC. SR141716A, a potent and selective antagonist of the brain cannabinoid receptor. FEBBE Lett. 1994; 350:240–44.

26. Barg,J, Fride,E, levy, R, Matus-Leibovitch, N, Heldman,E, Bayewitch, M, Mechoulam, R, Vogel, Z, Cannabinomimetic behavorial effects of and adenylate cyclase inhibition by two new endogenous anandamides. Eur J Pharmacol. 1995; 287:145–52.

27. Cravatt,BF, Prospero-Garcia,O, Siuzdak, G, Gilula, NB, Henriksen, SJ, Boger, DL, Lerner, RA, Chemical characteristics of a family of brain-lipids that induce sleep. Science. 1995; 268:1506–1509.

28. Sheskim, T, Hanus, L, Slager,J, Vogel,Z, Mechoulam, R. Structural requirements for binding of anandamide-type compounds to the brain cannabinoid receptor. J Med Chem 1997; 40:659–667.

29. Maurelli, S, Bisogno, T, De Perocelli,L, Luccia, A, Marino,G, Marzo,V. Two novel classes of neuroactive fatty acid amides are substrates for mouse neuroblastoma anandamide amidohydrolase. FEBS lett. 1995; 377:82–86.

30. DiMarzo, V, Fontana, A, Cadas, H, Schinelli, S, Cimino, G, Schwartz, JC, Piomelli,D. Formation and inactivation of endogenous cannabinoid anandamide in central neurons, Nature. 1994; 372:686–691.

31. Shen, M, Piser,TM, Seybold,VS, Thayer, SA. Cannabinoid receptor agonists inhibit glutamateric synaptic transmission in rat hippocampal cultures. J Neurosci. 1996; 16:4322–34.

32. Chan, PKY, Chan, SCY, Yung,WH. Presynaptic inhibition of GABAergic inputs to rat substantia nigra pars reticulate neurons by a cannabinoid agonist. NeuroReport. 1998; 9:671–5.

33. Hoffman, AF, Lupica,CR. Mechanisms of cannabinoid inhibition of GABA(A) synaptic transmission in the hippocampus. J. Neurosci. 2000; 20:2470–79.

34. Takahinshi,KA, Linden, DJ. Cannabinoid receptor modulation of synapses received by cerebellar purkinje cells. J Neurophysiol. 2000; 83:1167–80.

35. Heyser, CJ, Hampson, RE, Deadwyler, SA. Effects of delta-9- tetrahydrocannabinol on delayed match to sample performance in rats: alterations in short-term memory associated with changes in task specific firing

in hippocampal cells. J Pharmacol Exp Ther. 1993; 264:294–307.

36. Lichtman, AH, Dimen, KR. Martin, BR. Systemic or intrahippocampal cannabinoid administration impairs spatial memory in rats> Psychopharmacol (Berl). 1995; 119: 282–290.

37. Hampson,RE, Deadwyler, SA. Cannabinoids, hippocampal function and memory. Life Sci. 1999; 65:715–723.

38. Kim, DJ, Thayer, SA. Activation of CB1 cannabinoid receptors inhibits neurotransmitter release from identified synaptic sites in rat hippocampal cultures. Brain Res. 2000; 852: 398–405.

39. Katona,I, Sperlagh, B, Sik, A, Kafalvi, A, Vizi, ES, Mackie, K, Freund, TF. Presynaptically located CB1 cannabinoid receptors regulate GABA release fron axon terminals of specific hippocampal Interneurons. J Neurosci. 1999; 19:4544–4558.

40. Irving, AJ, Coutts, AA, Harvey, J, Raee, MG, Mackie,K, Bewick, GS, Pertwee, RG. Functional expression of cell surface cannabinoid CB1 receptors on presynaptic inhibitory terminals in cultured ratt hippocampal neurons. Neurosci. 2000; 98:253–262.

41. Pertwee, RG. Cannabinoid receptors and pain. Prog. Neurobiol. 2001; 63:569–611.

42. Friedman, HV, Bresler, T, Garner, CC, Ziv, NE. Assembly of new individual excitatory synapses: time course and temporal order of synaptic molecular recruitment. Neuron. 2000; 27:57–69.

43. Marsiconi, G, Wotjak, CT, Azad, SC, Bisogno,T, Rammes, G, Cascio, MG, Hermann, H, Tang, J, Hofmann, C, Zieglgansberger, DiMarco, V, Lutz,B. The endogenous cannabinoid system controls extinction of aversive memories. Nature. 2002; 418:530–4.

44. Falls, WA, Miserendino, MJ, Davis, M. Extinction of fear-potentiated startle: blockade by infusion of an NMDA antagonist into the amygdala. J Neurosci. 1992; 12: 854–863.

45. Ishac, EJN, Jiang, L, Lake, KD, Varga, K, Abood, ME, Kunos, G. Inhibition of exocytotic noradrenaline release by presynaptic cannabinoid CB1 receptors on peripheral sympathetic nerves. Br J Pharmacol. 1996; 118:2023–2028.

46. Wickens, AP, Pertwee, RG. Delta-9-Tetrahydrocannabinol and anandamide enhance the ability of muscimol to induce cataplexy in the globus pallidis of rats. Eur J PharmaCOL. 1993; 250:205–8.

47. Romero,J, Garcia-Palomero,E, Fernandez-uiz,JJ, Ramos, JA. Involvement of GABA(B) receptors in the motor inhibition produced by agonists of brain cannabinoid receptors. Behav Pharmacol. 1996; 7: 299–302.

48. Bilkei-Gorzo,A, Erk, S, Schurman,B, Mauer, D, Michel,K, Boecker,H, Scheef, L, Walter, H, Zimmer, A. Dynorphins Regulate Fear Memory: from mice to men. J Neurosci. 2012; 32(27): 9335–9343.

49. Zygmunt,PM, Petersson,J, Anderson, DA, Chuang,H-H, Sorgard, M, DiMarzo V, Julius,D, Hogestatt, ED. Vanilloid receptors on sensory nerves mediate the vasodilator action of anandamide. Nature. 1999; 400; 452–7.

50. Ledent, C, Valverde, O, Cossu, G, Petitet, F, Aubert, J-F, Beslot, F, Bohme, G, Imperato, A, Pedrazzini, T, Roques, BP, Vassart, G, Fratta, W, Parmentier, M. Unresponsiveness to cannabinoids and reduced additive Effects of Opiates in CB1 Receptor Knockout Mice. Science. 1999; 283:401–4.

51. Straiker,A, Stella, N, Piomelli, D, Mackie,K, Karten, HJ, Maguire, G. Cannabinoid CB1 receptors and ligands in vertebrate retina: localization and function of an endogenous signaling system. PNAS. 1999; 96:14565–70.

52. Schmid, PC, Krebsbach, RJ, Perry, SR, Dettmer, TM, Massen, JL, Schmidt, HHo. Occurance and postmortem generation of anandamide and other long-chain N-acylethanolamides in mammalian brain. FEBS Lett. 1995; 375117–120.

53. Kempe, K, Hsu, FF, Bohrer, A, Turk, J. Isotope dilution mass spectrometric measurements indicate that arachidonylethanolamine, the proposed endogenous ligand of the cannabinoid receptor, accumulates in the rat brain tissue post mortem but is contained at low levels in or absent from fresh tissue. J Biol Chem. 1996; 271:17287–17295.

54. Felder,CC, Nielsen, A, Briley, EM, Palkovitis, M, Priller, J, Axelrod, J, Nguyen, DN,

Richardson, JM,, Riggin, RM, Koppel, GA, Paul, SM, Becker, GW. Isolation and measurement of the endogenous cannabinoid receptor agonist, anandamide, in the brain and peripheral tissues of human and rat. FEBS Lett. 1996; 393:231–235.

55. Schmid, HHO, Schmid, PC, Natajaran, V. N-acylated glycerolphospholipids and their derativites. Prog Lipid Res. 1990; 29:1–43.

56. Schmid, PC, Reddy, PV, Natarajan, V Schmid HHO. Metabolism of N-acylethanolamine phospholipids by a mammalian phosphodiesterase of the phospholipase D type. J Biol Chem. 1983; 258:9302–9306.

57. Weidenfeld, J, Feldman, S, Mechoulam, R. Effects of the brain constituent anandamide, a cannabinoid receptor agonist, on the hypothalamic-pituitary-adrenal axis in the rat. Neuroendocrinology. 1994; 59: 110–112.

58. Wenger, T, Toth, BE, Martin, BR. Effects of anandamide(endogen cannabinoid) on anterior pituitary hormone secretion in adult ovariectomized rats. Life Sci. 1995; 56:2057–2063.

59. Giannikou, P, Yiannakakis, N, Frangkakis, G, Probonas, K, Wenger, T, Anandamide(endogen cannabinoid) decreases serum prolactin level in pregnant rats. Neuroendocrinol Lett. 1995; 17:281–287.

60. Bisogno,T, Maurelli,S, Melck, D, DePetrocellis, L, DiMarzo,V. Biosynthesis, uptake and degredation of anandamide and palmitoylethanolamide in leukocytes. J Biol Chem. 1997; 272:3315–3323.

61. Facci, L, DalToso, R, Romanello, S, Buriani, A, Skapper, SD, Leon A. Mast cells express a peripheral cannabinoid receptor with differential sensitivity to anandamide and palmitoylethanolamide. Proc Natl Acad Sci USA. 1995; 92: 3376–3380.

62. Schwarz, H, alanco, FJ, Lotz, M. Anandamide, an endogenous cannabinoid receptor agonist inhibits lymphocyte proliferation and induces apoptosis. J Neuroimmunol. 1994; 55:107–115.

63. Mazzari, S, Canella, R, Peterelli, L, Marcolongo, G, Leon, A. N-(2-hydroxyethyl) hexadecanamide id orally active in reducing edema formation and inflammatory hyperalgesia by down-regulating mast cell

activation. Eur J Pharmacol. 1996; 300:227–36.

64. Gerard, CM, Mollereau, C, Vassart, G, Parimentier, M. Nucleotide sequence of a human cannabinoid receptor cDNA. Nucleic Acids Res. 1990; 18:7142–134.

65. Sugiura, T, Kondo, S, Sukagawa,A, Tonegawa, T, Nakane, S, Yamashita, A, Waku, K. Enzymatic synthesis of anandamide, an endogenous receptor ligand, through N-acylphosphatidyloethanolamine patheay in testis: involvement od Ca2+ dependent transacylase and phosphodiesterase activities. Biochem Biophys Res Comm. 1996; 218:113–117.

66. Pertwee,RG, Joeadigwe,G, Hawksworth, GM. Further evidence for the presence of cannabinoid CB1 receptors in mouse vas deferens. Eur J Pharmacol. 1996; 296:169–172.

67. Chang, MC, Berkery, D, Schuel, R, Laychock, SG, Zimmerman, AM, Zimmerman, S, Schuel, H. Evidence for a cannabinoid receptor in sea urchin sperm and its role in blockade of the acrosome reaction. Mol Reprod Develop. 1993; 36:507–16.

68. Schuel, H, Berkery, D. Chang, MC, Zimmerman, AM, Zimmerman, S. Reduction of the fertilizing capacity of the sea urchin sperm by cannabinoids derived from marijuana: Inhibition of the acrosome reaction induced by egg jelly. Mol Repro Develop. 1991; 29:51–9.

69. Schuel, H, Goldstein, E, Mechoulam, R, Zimmerman, AM, Zimmerman, S. Anandamide9arachiodynlethanolamide), a brain cannabinoid receptor agonist, reduces sperm fertilizing capacity in sea urchins by inhibiting the acrosome reaction. Proc Natl Acad Sci USA. 1994; 91:7678–7682.

70. Bisogno, T, Ventrigila, M, Mosca, M, Milone, A, Cimino, G, DiMarzo, V. Occurrence and metabolism of anandamide and related acylethanolamides in ovaries of the sea urchin Paracentrotus lividus. Biochem Biophys Acta. 1997; 1345:338–348.

71. Paria, BC, Das, SK, Dey, SK. The perimplantation embryo is a target for cannabinoid ligand-receptor signaling. Proc Natl Acad Sci USA. 1995; 92:9460–9464.

72. Paria, BC, Deutsch, DD, Dev, SK. The uterus is a potential site for anandamide synthesis and

hydrolysis: differential profiles of anandamide synthase and hydrolase activities in the mouse uterus during the periimplantation period. Mol Repr Develop. 1996; 45:183–192.

73. Maccarrone, M., Dainese, E., Oddi, S. Intracellular trafficking of anandamide: new concepts for wsignaling. Trend Biochem Sci. 2010; 35:601–8. Doi 10.1016/j.tibs.2010.05.008.

74. Muccioli, G. G. Endocannabinoid biosynthesis and inactivation, from simple to complex. Drug Discov. Today. 2010; 15:474–83. doi. 10.1016/j.drudis.2010.03.007

75. Okamato Y., Tsuboi, K., Ueda, N. Enzymatic formation of anandamide. Vitam Norm. 2009; 81:1–24 doi. 10.1016/s0083-6729(09)81001-7

76. McKinney, M. K., Cravatt, B. F. Structure and function of fatty acid amide hydrolase, Ann Rev Biochem. 2005; 74:411–32 doi. 10.1146/annurev.biochem.74.082803.133450

77. Udea, N., Tsuboi, K., Uyama, T., Ohnishi, T, Biosynthesis and degradation of the endocannabinoid 2-arachidonylglycerol. Biofactors. 2011; 37:1–7. doi.10.1002/biof.131

78. Dinh, T.P., Freund, T.,F. Piomelli, D. A role for monoglyceride lipase in 2-arachidonylglycerol inactivation. Chem Phys Lipids. 2002; 121:149–58 doi.10.1016/S0009-3084(02)00150-0

79. Van Sickle, M. D., Duncan, M., Kingsley, P. J., Mouihate, A., Urbani, P., Mackie, K., Stella, N., Makriyannis A., et al.Identification and functional characterization of brainstem cannabinoid CB2 receptors. Science. 2005; 310:329–32 . doi. 10.1126/science.1115740

80. Viscomi, M.T., Oddi, S. Latini, L., Pasquariello, N., Florenzano, F., Bernardi, G., Molinari, M., Maccarrone, M. Selective CB2 receptor agonism protects central neurons from remote axotomy-induced apoptosis through the P13K. Akt pathway. J. Neurosci. 2009; 29:4564–70. doi. 10.1523/jneurosci.0786–09.2009.

81. Pertwee, R.G. GPR55: a new member of the cannabinoid receptor clan? Br J Pharmacol. 2007; 152:984–6. doi. 10.1038/sj.bjp.0707464

82. Ryberg, E., Larsson, N., Sjogren, S., Hjorth, S., Hermansson, N. O., Leonova, J., Elebring, T., Nilsson, K., Drmota, T., Greasley, P.J. The orphan receptor GPR55 is a novel cannabinoid receptor. Br J Pharmacol. 2007; 152:1092–1101.doi.10.1038/sj.bjp.0707460

83. Lauckner, J. E., Jensen, J. B., Chen, H.Y., Lu, H.C., Hille, B., Mackie, K. GPR55 is a cannabinoid receptor that increases intracellular calcium and inhibits M current. Proc. Natl. Acad. Sci USA. 2008; 105:2699–2704 doi.10.1073/pnas.0711278105

84. DiMarzo, V., DePetrocellis, L. Endocannabinoid as regulators of transient receptor potential(TRP) channels: a further opportunity to develop new endocannabinoid-based therapeutic drugs. Curr. Med. Chem. 2010; 17:1430–49

85. Pistis, M., Melis, M. From surface to nuclear receptors: the endocannabinoid family extends its assets. Curr. Med. Chem. 2010; 17:1450–1467.

86. Bari, M., Battista, N., Fezza, F., Finazzi Agro, A., Maccarrone, M. Lipid rafts control signaling of type-1 cannabinoid receptors in neuronal cells. Implications for anandamide-induced apoptosis. J Biol. Chem. 2005; 280:12212–12220 doi.10.1074/jbc.M411642200

87. Sarnataro, D., Grimaldi, C., Pisanti, S., Gazzerro, P., Laezza, C., Zurolo, C., Bifulco, M. Plasma membrane and lysosomal localization of CB1 cannabinoid receptors are dependent on lipid rafts and regulated by anandamide in human breast cancer cells. FEBS Lett. 2005; 579:6343–6349.

88. Dainese,E., Oddi, S., Bari, M., Maccarrone, M. Modulation of the endocannabinoid system by lipid rafts. Curr. Med. Chem. 2007; 14:2702–2715.

89. Hendstrige, C. M., Balenga, N.A., Ford, L.A., Ross, R.A., Waldhoer, M., Irving,A.J. The GPR55 ligand L-alphalysophitadylinositol promotes RhoA-dpendent Ca2+ signaling and NFAT activation. FASEB J. 2009; 23:183–93. Doi.10.1096/fj.08–108670

90. Oka, S., Nakajima, K., Yamashita, A., Kishimoto, S., Sugiura,T. Identification od GPR55 as a lysophosphatidylinositol receptor. Biochem. Biophys. Res. Commun. 2007; 362:928–34 doi. 10.1016/j.bbrc.2007.08.078

91. Oka, S., Toshida,T., Maruyama, K., Nakajima, K., Yamashita,A., Sugiura,T. 2-Arachidonoyl-sn-glycero-3-phosphoinositol: possible natural ligand for GPR55. J.Biochem. 2009; 145:13–20 doi.10.1093/jb/mvn136

92. Lanzaflame, A.A., Guida, E., Christopoulos, A. Effects of anandamide on the binding and signaling properties of M1 muscarinic acetylcholine receptors. Biochem. Pharmacol. 2004; 68: 2207–2219 doi.10.1016/j.bcp.2004.08.005

93. Manzaranes, J., Corchero, J., Romero, J., Fernandez-Ruiz, J.J., Ramos,J.A., Fuentes, J.A. Pharmacological and biochemical interactions between opioids and cannabinoids. Trends Pharmacol. Sci.1999; 20:287–294 doi. 10.1016/S0165-6147(99)01339-5

94. Beinfeld, M.C., Connolly,K. Activation of CB1 cannabinoid receptors in rat hippocampus slices inhibits potassium-evoked cholecystokinin release, a possible mechanism contributing to the spatial memory defects produced by cannabinoids. Neurosci. Lett. 2001; 301:69–71 doi. 10.1016/S0304-3940(01)01591-9

95. Ghozland,S., Mathes,H,W., Simonin,F., Filliol, D., Kieffer, B.L., Maldonado,R. Motivational effects of cannabinoids are mediated by mu-opioid and kappa receptors. J Neurosci. 2002; 22:1146–1154

96. Lopez-Moreno, J. A., Gonzales-Cuevas, G., Moreno,G., Navarro,M. The pharmacology of the endocannabinoid system: functional and structural interactions with other neurotransmitter systems and their repercissions in behavorial addiction. Addict. Biol. 2008; 13:160–187 doi. 10.1111/j.1369-1600.2008.00105.x.

97. Ligresti, A., Petrosino, S., DiMarzo,V. From endocannabinoid profiling to "endocannabinoid therapeutics". Curr. Opin. Chem. Biol. 2009; 13:21–31

98. doi.10.1016/j.cbpa.2009.04.615

99. Parmentier-Batteur, S., Jin, K., Mao, X. O.,Xie, L., Greenberg, D.A. Increased severity of stroke in CB1 cannabinoid receptor knock-out mice. J. Neurosci. 2002; 22:9771–9975.

100. Nagayama, T., Sinor, A.D., Simon, R.P., Chen, J., Graham, S.H., Jin, K., Greenberg, D.A.Cannabinoids and neuroprotection in global and focal cerebral ischemia and in neuronal cultures. J. Neurosci. 1999; 19:2987–2995.

101. Alonso-Alconada, D., Alvarez, F.J., Alvarez, A., Mielgo, V.E., Goni-de-Cerio, F., Rey-Santano, M.C., Caballero, A., Martinez-Orgado, J., Hilario, E. The cannabinoid recepror agonist WIN55,212–2 reduces the initial cerebral damage after hypoxic-ischemic injury in fetal lambs. Brain Res. 2010; 1362:150–159 doi. 10.1016/j.brainres.2010.09.050

102. Cunha, P., Romao, A.M., Mascarenhas-Melo, F., Teizeira, H. M., Reis,F. Endocannabinoid system in cardiovascular disorders- new pharmacotherapeutic opportunities. J. Pharm. Bioallied Sci. 2011; 3:350–360 doi.10.4103/0975-7406.84435

103. Zhang, M., Adler, M.W., Abood, M.E., Ganea, D., Jallo, J., Tuma, R.F. CB2 receptor activation attenuates microcirculatory dysfunction during cerebral ischemic/reperfusion injury. Microvasc. Res. 2009; 78:86–94 doi.10.1016/j.mvr.2009.03.005

104. Zhang, M., Martin, B.R., Adler, M.W., Razdan, R.K., Jallo, J.I., Tima, R.F. Cannabinoid CB(2) receptor activation decreases cerebral infarction in a mouse focal ischemic/reperfusion model. J. Cereb. Blood Flow Mtab. 2007; 27:1387–1396 doi. 10.1038/sj.jcbfm.9600447

105. Hanus, L., Breuer,A., Tchillibon, S., Shiloah, S., Goldberg, D., Horowitz, M., Pertwee, R.G., Ross, R.A., Mechoulam, R., Fride,E. HU-308: a specific agonist for CB2, a peripheral cannabinoid receptor. Proc. Natl. Acad. Sci. USA 1999; 96:14228–14233 doi.10.1073/pnas.96.25.14228

106. Yao, B.B., Mukherjee, S., Fan, Y., Garrison, T.R., Daza, A. V., Grayson, G.K., Hooker, B.A., Dart, M.J., Sullivan, J.P., Meyer, M.D. In vitro pharmacological characterization of AM1241: a protean agonist at the cannabinoid CB2 receptor? Br. J. Pharmacol. 2006; 149:145–154 doi.10.1038/sj.bjp.0706838

107. Centonze,D., Finazzi Argo, A., Bernardi, G., Maccarrone, M. The endocannabinoid system

in targeting inflammatory neurodegenerative diseases. Trends Pharmacol. 2007; 28: 180–187 doi. 10.1016/j.tips.2007.02.004

108. DiMarzo,V. CB(1) receptor antagonism: biological basis for metabolic effects. Drug Discov. Today 2008; 13:1026–1041 doi.10.1016/j.drudis.2008.09.001

109. Christopoulou, F.D., Kiortsis, D. N. An overview of the metabolic effects of rimonabant in randomized controlled trials: potential for other cannabinoid 1 receptor blockers in obesity. J. Clin. Pharm. Ther. 2011; 36:10–18 doi. 10.1111/j.1365-2710.2010.01164

110. Bari, M., Battista, N., Pirazzi, V., Maccarrone, M. The manifold actions of endocannabinoids on female and male reproductive events. Front. Biosci. 2011; 16:198–516 doi. 10.2741/3701

ANXIETY

1. Akirav, I. Role of the Endocannabinoid System in Anxiety and Stress-Related Disorders, http://www.interchopen.com/books/anxiety-disorders/role-of-the-endocannabinoid-system-in-anxiety-and-stress-related-disorders1.

2. Marsciano, G., Wotjak, C.T., Azad, S.C., Bisogno,T., Rammes, G., Cascio, .., et al. The endogenous cannabinoid system controls extinction of aversive memories. Nature 2002; 418(6897):530–534.

3. Herkenham, M., Lynn, A.B., Johnson, M.R., Melvin, L.S., deCosta, B.R.Rice, K.C. Characterization and localization of cannabinoid receptors in rat brain: A quantitative in vitro autoradiograpic study. J Neurosci 1991; 11(2): 563–583.

4. Freund, T.F., Katona,I., Pimelli,D. Role of the endogenous cannabinoids in synaptic signaling. Physiol Rerv 2003; 83(3): 1017–1066.

5. Pazos,M.R., Benito, C., Tolon, R.M.,Romero, J. Functional neuroanatomy of the endocannabinoid system. Pharm Biochem and Behavior 2005; 81(2):239–247.

6. Svizenska, I., Dubovi, P., Sulcova, A. Cannabinoid receptors 1 and 2 (CB1 and CB2), their distribution, ligands and functional involvement in nervous system structures—a short review. Pharm Biochem and Behav. 2008; 90(4):501–511.

7. Breivogel,C.S., Sim-Selly Basic neuroanatomy and neuropharmacology of cannabinoids. Intl Rev Psych 2009; 21(2):113–121.

8. Viveros, M.,Marco, E.M., File, S.E, Endocannabinoid system and stress and anxiety responses. Pharm Biochem and Behav2005; 81(2): 331–342.

9. Laviolette,S.R., Grace, A.A.. Cannabinoids potentiate learning plasticity in neurons of the medial prefrontal cortex through basolateral amygdala inputs. J Neurosci. 2006; 26(24): 6458–6468.

10. Lavioletti,S.R., Grace,A.A. The roles of cannabinoid and dopamine receptor systems in neural emotional learning circuits: Implications for schizophrenia and addiction. Cellular and Molecular Life Sciences 2006; 63(14):1597–1613.

11. Gorzalka, R., Hill, M.N.,Hillard, C.J. Regulation of endocannabinoid signaling by stress: Implications for stress related affective disorders. Neurosci and Biobehavorial Rev. 2008; 32(6):1152–1160.

12. Ganor-Elazar, F., Akirav, I. Cannabinoid receptor activation in the basolateral amygdala blocks the effects of stress on the conditioning and extinction of inhibitory avoidance. J. Neurosci 2009; 29(36):11078–11088.

13. Lutz, B. Endocannabinoid signals in the control of emotion. Curr Opinion in Pharmacology 2009; 9(1): 46–52.

14. Hill, M.N., Gorzalka, B.B. The endocannabinoid system and the treatment of mood and anxiety disorders CNS&Neurologic Disorders-Drug Targets(Formerly Current Drug Targets) 2009; 8(6)451–458.

15. Parolaro,D.,Realini,N., Vigano,D., Rubino, T. The endocannabinoid system and psychiatric disorders Experimental Neurology 2010; 224(1):3–14.

16. Akirav,I., Maroun,M. The role of the medial prefrontal cortex-amygdala circuit in stress effects on the extinction of fear. Neural Plasticity, 2007, 30873.

17. Jankord, R., Herman, J.P. Limbic regulation of Hypothalamo-Pituitary-Adrenocortical

function during acute and chronic stress. Ann New York Acad of Sciences 2008; 1148(1):64–73.

18. Joels, M., Baram, T.Z. The neuro-symphony of stress. Nature Review Neuroscience 2009; 10(6): 459–66.

19. Viveros, M., Marco, E.,Llorente, R. Lopez-Gallardo,M. Endocannabinoid system and synaptic plasticity: Implications fo emotional response. Neural Plasticity 2007; 52908

20. Taber, K.H., Hurley, R.A. Endocannabinoids: stress, anxiety and fear, J Neuropsychiatry and Clin Neurosci. 2009; 21(2):108–113.

21. Shin,L.M., Liberzon, I. The neurocircuitry of fear, stress and anxiety disorders. Neuropsychopharmacology 2010; 35(1):169–191. doi.10.1038/npp.2009.83.

22. DeKloet, E.R.,Joels, M. Stress and the brain: From adaptation to disease. Nature Reviews Neuroscience. 2005; 6(6):463–75.

23. McEwen, B.S., Gould, E. adrenal steroid influences on the survival of hippocampal neurons. Biochem Pharmacol 1990; 40: 2393–2402.

24. McEwen, B.S. Stress and hippocampal plasticity. Ann. Review of Neurosci. 1999; 22(1):105–22.

25. Sapolsky, R.M. Why stress is bad for your brain. Science 1996; 273(5276):749–50.

26. Meaney,M.J.Maternal care, gene expression and the transmission of individual differences in stress reactivity across generations. Neuroscience 2001,2411611192

27. Bremner, J.D., Randall,P., Scott, T.M., Bronen, R.A., Seibyl, J.P.,et al.MRI-based measurement of hippocampal volume in patients with combat-related posttraumatic stress disorder.Am J Psychiatry 1995; 152(7):973–81.

28. Sheline, Y.I., Sanghavi, M., Mintum, M.A., Gado, M.H. Depression duration but not age predicts hippocampal volume loss in medically healthy women with recurrent major depression. J. Neurosci.1999; 19(12):5034–43.

29. Woon, F.L., Hedges, D.W. Hippocampal and amygdala volumes in children and adults with childhood maltreatment-related posttraumatic stress disorder: A meta-analysis. Hippocampus 2008; 1898):729–36.

30. Pitman, R.K., Gilbertson, M.W., Gurvits, T.V., May, F.S., Lasko, N.B. Metzger, L.J. et al. Clarifying the origin of biological abnormalities in PTSD through the study of identical twins discordant for combat exposure. Ann of New York Academy of Sciences 2006; 1071(1): 242–54.

31. Davis, M., The role of the amygdala in fear and anxiety. Ann. Review of Neuroscience 1992; 15(1):353–375.

32. LeDoux, J. The amygdala. Current Biology: CB 2007; 17(20): R868874

33. McDonald, A.J. Cortical pathways to the mammalian amygdala. Progress in Neurobiology. 1998; 55(3):257–332.

34. Pitkanen,A., Pikkarainen, M., Nurminen, N., Ylinen,A. reciprocal connections between the amygdala and the hippocampal formation, perirhinal cortex, and postrhinal cortex in rat: A review. Annals of the New York Academy of Sciences. 2000; 911(1): 369–391.

35. Goldman-Rakic, P.S>, Cools, A., Srivastava, K. The prefrontal landscape: Implications of functional architecture for understanding human memtation and the central executive (and discussion). Philosophical Transactions: Biological Sciences. 1996; 351(1346): 1445–53.

36. Rolls, E.T., Everitt, B. The orbitofrontal cortex (and discussion) Philosophical Transactions of the Royal Society off London, Series B: Biological Sciences. 1996; 351(1346):1433.

37. Trembley, L., Schultz, W. Relative reward preference in primate orbitofrontal cortex. Nature 1999; 398(6729):704–8.

38. Bush, G., Luu, P., Posner,I. Cognitive and emotional influences in anterior cingulate cortex. Trends in Cognitive Science.2000; 4(6):215–22.

39. Miller, E.K., Cohen, J.D. An integrative theory of prefrontal cortex function. Annual Review of Neuroscience. 2001; 24(1):167–202.

40. Robbins, T.W. Chemistry of the mind: neurochemical modulation of prefrontal cortical function. The J. of Comparative Neurology.2005; 493(1):140–146.

41. Holmes, A., Wellman, C.L. Stress –induced prefrontal organization and executive function in rodents. Neuroscience & Behavorial Reviews, 2009; 33(6):773–83.

42. Cahill,L., Haier, R.J., Fallon, J., Alkire, M.T., Tang, C., Keator, D., et al. Amygdala activity at encoding correlated with long-term, free recall of emotional information. Proceedings of the National Academy of Sciences, USA. 1996; 93(15):8016–8021.

43. Canali,T., Zhao,Z., Brewer, J., Gabrieli, J.D.E., Cahill, L. Event-related activation in the human amygdala associates with later memory for individual emotional experience. J. of Neuroscience. 2000; 20: RC9915

44. Richter-Levin,G., Akirav,I. Emotional tagging of memory formation—in the search for neural mechanisms. Brain Research Reviews. 2003; 43(3):247–256.

45. Joels, M., Karst,H., Alfarez,D. Heine, V.M., Qin, Y., Reil,E. Effects of chronic stress on structure and cell function in rat hippocampus and hypothalamus. Stress: The International ajournal on the BIOLOGY OF stress. 2004; 7(4):221–231.

46. McGaugh, J.L. The amygdala modulates the consolidation of memories of emotionally arousing experiences. Annu Rev. Neuroscience. 2004; 27128

47. Phelps, E.A. Human emotion and memory: Interactions of the amygdala and hippocampal complex. Current Opinion in Neurobiology. 2004; 14(2): 198–202.

48. Vianna, M.R., Coitinho, A.S., Izquierdo,I. Role of the hippocampus and amygdala in the extinction of fear motivated learning. Current Neurovascular Research. 2004; 1(1):55–60.

49. Diamond, D.M., Park, C.R., Campbell, A.M., Woodson, J.C. Competetive interactions between endogenous LTD AND ltp in the hippocampus underlie the storage of emotional memories and stress-induced amnesi. Hippocampus.2005; 15(8):1006–1025.

50. Willner, P., Muscat, R., Papp,M. Chronic mild stress-induced anhedonia: A realistic animal model of depression. Neuroscience& Biobehavorial Reviews.1992; 16(4):525–534.

51. Zangen,A., Nakash,R., Overestreet, D.H., Yadid, G. Association between depressive behavior and absent serotonin-dopamine interaction in the nucleus accimbens. Paychopharamacologia. 2001; 155(4): 434–439.

52. Nestler, E.J., Barrot, M., DiLeone, R.J., Eisch,A.J., Gold, S.J., Monteggia, L.M. Neurobiology of dwpression. Neuron.2002; 34(1):13–25.

53. Seamans, J.K., Phillips, .G. Selective memory impairments produced by transient lidocaine-induced lesions of the nucleus accumbens in rats. Behavorial Neuroscience.1994; 108(3):456–468.

54. Setlow, B., Roozenthal,B., McGaugh,J>L> Involvement of a basolateral amygdala complez-nucleus accumbens pathway in glucocorticoid-induced modulation of memory consolidation. European Journal of Neuroscience. 2000; 12(1):367–375.

55. Reynolds, S.M., Berridge, K.C. Positive and negative motivation in nucleus accumbens shell: Bivalent rostrocaudal gradients for GABA-elicited eating,taste"liking"/"disliking" reactions, place preference/avoidance, and fear. The Journal of Neuroscience.2002; 22(16):7308–7320.

56. Mogenson,G.J., Jones, D.L., Yim, C.Y. From motivation to action: Functional interface between the limbic system and the motor system. Progress in Neurobiology.1980; 14(2–3):69–97.

57. Petrovich, G., Risold, P., Swanson, L. Organization of projections from the basomedial nucleus of the amygdala: A PHAL study in the rat. The Journal of Comparative Neurology.1996; 374(3):387–420.

58. Groenewegen, H., der Zee,E., Te,A., Korschot, M., Witter,A. Organization of the projections from the subiculum to the ventral striatum in the rat. A study using anterograde transport of phaseolus vulgaris leucoagglutin. Neuroscience.1987; 23(1):103–120.

59. Meredith,G., Wouterlood, F., Pattiselanno,A. Hippocampal fibers make synaptic contacts with glutamate decarbylase-immunoreactive neurons in the rat nucleus accumbens. Brain Research. 1909; 513(2):329–334.

60. Nauta, W., Smith,G., Faull,R., Domesick,V.B. Efferent connections and nigral afferents of the nucleus accumbens septi in the rat. Neuroscience. 1978; 3(4–5):385–401.

61. Rodriguez de Fonseca,F., Carrera, M.R.A., Navarro,M., Koob, G.F., Weiss, F. Activation of corticotrophin-releasing factor in the limbic system during cannabinoid withdrawl. Science. 1997; 276(5321):2050–2054.

62. Scherma,M., Medalie,J., Fratta, W., Vadivel, S.K., Makriyannis, A., Piomelli, D., et al. The endogenous cannabinoid anandamide has effects on motivation and anxiety that are revealed by fatty acid amide hydrolase (FAAH) inhibition. Neuropharmacology2008; 54(1):129–140.

63. Lafenetre,P., Chaouloff, F., Marsicano, G. The endocannabinoid system in the processing of anxiety and fear and how CB1 receptors may modulate fear extinction. Pharmacologial Research. 2007; 56(5):367–381.

64. Hall, W., Solowjj, N. Adverse effects of cannabis. The Lancet. 1998; 352(9140):1611–1616.

65. Linszen, D., van Amelsvoort, T. Cannabis and psychosis: an update on course and biologic plausible mechanisms. Current Opinions in Psychiatry. 2007; 20(2):116–20.

66. Rubino, T. Role in anxiety behavior of the endocannabinoid system in the prefrontal cortex. Cerebral Cortex.2008; 18(6):1292–1301.

67. Patel, S., Hillard,C.J., Pharmacological evaluation of cannabinoid receptor ligands in a mouse model of anxiety: Further evidenxce for an anxiolytic role for endogenous cannabinoid signaling. J of Pharmacology and Experimental Therapeutics. 2006; 318(1): 304–311.

68. Rausch,S.L., Shin,L.M., Phelps, E.A. Neurocircuitry models of posttramatic stress disorder and extinction: Human neuroimaging research-past, present and future. Biological Psychiatry. 2006; 60(4):376–382.

69. Arenos, J.D., Musty, R.E., Bucci,D.J. Blockade of cannabinoid CB1 receptors alters contextual learning and memory. European Journal of Pharmacology. 2006; 539(3): 177–183.

70. Reich, C.G., Mohammadi, M.H., Alger, B.E. Endocannabinoid modulation of fear responses; Learning and state-dependent effects. Journal of Psychopharmacology. 2008; 22(7): 769–777.

71. Abush, H., Akirav, I. Cannabinoids modulate hippocampal memory and plasticity. Hippocampus. 2010; 20(10): 1126–1138.

72. Charney, D.S., Deutch, A.Y., Krystal, J.H., Southwick, S.M., Davis, M.Psychobiologic mechanisms of posttraumatic stress disorder. Archives of General Psychiaty. 1993; 50(4):294–305

73. Wessa,M., Flor,H. Failure of extinction of fear responses in posttraumatic stress disorder: evidence for second order conditioning. American Journal of Psychiatry. 2007; 164(11): 1684–92.

74. Milad,M.R., Orr, S.P., Lasko, N.B., Chang,Y., Rauch, S.L., Pitman, R.K. Presence and acquired origin of reduced recall for fear extinction in PTSD: results of a twin study. Journal of Psychiatric Research. 2008; 42(7): 515–20.

75. Milad, M.R., Quirk, G.J. Neurons in medial prefrontal cortex signal memory for fear extinction. Nature. 2002; 420(6911):70–74.

76. Bouton, M.E., Westbrook, R.F., Corcoran, K.A., Maren, S. Contextual and temporal modulation of extinction: Behavorial and biological mechanisms. Biological Psychiatry. 2006; 60(4): 352–360.

77. Suzuki,A., Josselyn, S.A., Frankland, P.W., Masushige, S., Silva, A.J., Kida,S. Memory reconsolidation and extinction have distinct temporal and biochemical signatures. Journal of Neuroscience. 2004; 24(20):4787–4795.

78. Finn, D., Beckett, S., Richardson, D., Kendall, D., Marsden, C., Chapman,V. Evidence for differential modulation of conditioned aversion and sear-conditioned analgesia by CB1 receptors. European Journal of Neuroscience. 2004; 20(3):848–852.

79. Chhatwal,J.P., Myers, K.M., Ressler, K.J. Davis, M. Regulation of gephyrin and GABA receptor binding within the amygdala after fear acquisition and extinction. Journal of Neuroscience. 2005; 25(2): 502–506.

80. Lutz, B. The endocannabinoid system and extinction learning. Molecular Neurobiology. 2007; 36(1):92–101.

81. Niyuhire,F., Varvel,S.A., Thorpe, A.J., Stokes, R.J., Wiley, J.L., Lichtman, A.H. The disruptive effects of the CB1 receptor antagonist rimonabant on extinction learning

in mice are task specific. Psychopharmacology. 2007; 191(2):223–231.

82. Varvel,S. et al. Inhibition of fatty-acid amide hydrolase accelerates acquisition and extinction rates in a spatial memory task. Neuropsychopharmacology. 2007; 32(5):1032–1041.

83. Katona, I., RaNC, E.A., Acsady, L., Ledent, C., Mackie, K., Hajoa,N. et al. Distribution of CB1 cannabinoid receptors in the amygdala and their role in the control of GABAergic transmission. Journal of Neuroscience.2001; 21(23):9506–9518.

84. Kamprath, K., Marsicano,G., Tang, J., Monory,K., Bisogno, T., Marzo, V.D. et al. Cannabinoid CB1 receptor mediates fear extinction via habituation-like processes. Journal of Neuroscience. 2006; 26(25):6677–6686.

85. Pistis, M., Perra,S., Pillolla, G., Melis, M., Gessa, G.L., Muntoni, A.L. Cannabinoids modulate neuronal firing in the rat basolateral amygdala; Evidence for CB1 and non-CB1-mediated actions. Neuropharmacology. 2004; 46(1):115–125.

86. Patel, S., Roelke,C.T., Rademcher, D.J., Hillard, C.J. Inhibition of restraint stress-induced neural and behavorial activation by endogenous cannabinoid signaling. European Journal of Neuroscience. 2005; 21(4): 1057–1069

87. Finn, D.P. Endocannabinoid-mediated modulation of stress response: physiological and pathophysiological significance Immuniobiology. 2010; 215(8):629–46.

88. Pecoraro, N., Dallman, M.F., Warne, J.P., Ginsberg, A.B., Laugero, K.D., la Fleur, S.E. et al. From Malthus to motive: How the HPA axis engineers the phenotype, voking needs to wants. Progress in Neurobiology.2006; 79(5–6): 247–340.

89. Di Malcher-Lopez, S.R., Marcheselli, V.L., Bazam, N.G., Tasker, J.G. Rapid glucocorticoid-mediated endocannabinoid release and opposing regulation of glutamate and (gamma)-aminobutyric acid inputs to hypothalamic Magnocellular neurons. Endocrinology. 2005; 146(10):4292–4301.

90. Di Malcher-Lopez, S.R., Marcheselli, S.V.S., Weng, F.J., Stuart, C.T., Bazan, N.G., et al. Opposing crosstalk between leptin and glucocorticoids rapidly modulates synaptic excitation via endocannabinoid release. Journal of Neuroscience. 2006; 26(24):6643–6650.

91. Hohmann, A.G., Suplita, R.L., Bolton, N.M., Neely, M.H., Fegley, D., Mangieri, R., et al. An endocannabinoid mechanism for stress-induced analgesia. Nature. 2005; 435(7045):1108–1112.

92. Rademacher, D.J., Meier, S.E., Shi, L., Vanessa, H.W.S., Jarrahian, A., Hillard, C.J. Effects of acute and repeated restraint stress on endocannabinoid content in the amygdala, ventral striatum, and prefrontal cortex in mice. Neuropharmacology.2008; 54(1): 108–116.

93. Patel, S., Cravatt, B.F., Hillard, C.J. Synergistic interactions between cannabinoids and environmental stress in the activation of the central amygdala. Neuropsychopharamacology. 2004; 30(3):497–507.

94. Hill, M.N., McLaughlin,R.J., Morrish, A.C., Viau, V., Floresco, S.B., Hillard, C.J. et al. Suppression of amygdala endocannabinoid signaling by stress contributes to activation of the Hypothalamic-Pituitary-Adrenal axis. Neuropsychopharamacology. 2009; 34(13): 2733–2745.

95. Viveros,M., Marco, E.M., File, S.F. Endocannabinoid system and stress and anxiety responses. Pharmacology Biochemistry and Behavior. 2005; 81(2): 331–342

96. Chang, L., Chronicle, E.P. Functional imaging studies in cannabis users. The Neuroscientists.2007; 13(5): 422–432.

97. Bambico, F.R., Katz,N., Debonnel,G., Gobbi, G. Cannabinoids elicit antidepressant-like behavior and activate serotonergic neurons through the medal prefrontal cortex. Journal of Neuroscience.2007; 27(43): 11700–11711.

98. Moreira, F.A., Aguiar, D.C., Guimaraes, F.S. Anxyolytic-like effect of cannabinoids injected into the dorsolateral periaqueductal gray. Neuropharmacology. 2007; 52(3): 958–965.

99. Rubino, T. CB1 receptor stimulation in specific brain areas differently modulate anxiety-related behavior. Neuropharmacology. 2008; 54(1): 151–160.

100. Marsicano, G., Wojak, C.T., Azad, S.C., Bisogno,T., Rammes, G., Cascio, M.G., et al. The endogenous cannabinoid system controls extinction of aversive memories. Nature; 418(6897):530–534.

IMMUNE SYSTEM

1. Izzo, A.A., Borrelli, F., Capasso, R., DiMarzo, V., Mechoulam, R. Non-psychotrophic plant cannabinoids: new rherapeutic opportnunities from an ancient herb. Trends in Pharmacological Sci. 2009; 30:515–527 doi: 10.1016/j.tips.2009.07.006

2. Mechoulsm, R. Cannabidiol recent advances. Chem. Biodivers. 2007; 4:1678–1692

3. Carrier. E.J. Inhibition of an equilibrtative nucleoside transporter by cannabidiol: a mechanism of cannabidiol immuniosupression. Proc Natl. Acad. Sci. USA. 2006; 103:7895–7900.

4. McHugh, D., et al. Inhibition of human neutrophil chemotaxis by endogenous cannabinoids and phytocannabinoids: evidence for a site distinct from CB1 and CB2. Mol. Pharmacol. 2008; 73:441–450.

5. Jan, T.R., et. Al. Supressive effects of cannabidiol on antigen specific antibody production and functional activity of splenocytes in ovalbumin-sensitized BALB/c mice. Int. Immuniopharmacol. 2008; 7: 773–780

6. Jenny, M. et al. Delta9-tetrahydrocannabinol and cannabidiol modulate mitogen-induced tryptophan degredation and neopterin formation in peripheral blood mononuclear cells in vitro. J. Neuroimmunol. 2009; 207: 75–82

7. Lee, C.Y. et al. A comparative study on cannabidiol-induced apoptosis in murine thymocytes and EL-4 thymoma cells. Int. Immuniopharmacol. 2008; 8: 732–740.

8. Wu, H. Y., et al. Cannabidiol-induced a[poptosis in primary lymphocytes is associated with oxidative stress-dependent activation of capase-8. Toxicol. Appl. Pharmacol. 2008; 226:260–270.

9. Kaplan, B.L., et al The profile of immune modulation by cannabidiol (CBD) involves deregulation of nuclear factor of activated T-cells (NFAT). Biochem. Pharmacol. 2008; 76: 726–737.

10. Galiegue, S., etal. Expression of central and peripheral cannabinoid receptors in human immune tissues and leukocyte subpopulations. Eur. J. Biochem. 1995; 232:54–61.

11. Schatz, A.R., et al. Cannabinoid receptors CB1 and CB2: a characterization of expression and adenylate cyclase modulation within the immune system. Toxicol. Appl. Pharmacol. 1997; 142:278–287.

12. Nunez, E., et al. Cannabinoid CB2 receptors are expressed by perivascular microglial cells in the human brain: an immuniohistochemical study. Synapse. 2004; 53:208–213.

13. Ramirez, B.G. et al. Prevention of Alzheimer's disease pathology by cannabinoids: neuroprotection mediated by blockade of microglial activation. J. Neurosci. 2005; 25:1904–1913.

14. Cabral, G.A., Marciano-Cabral, F. Cannabinoid receptors in microglia of the central nervous system: immune functional relevance. J. Leukoc. Biol. 2005; 78: 1192–1197.

15. Fernandez-Ruis, J., et al. Cannabinoid CB2 receptor: a new target for controlling neural cell survival? Trends Pharmacol. Sci. 2007; 28:39–45.

16. Zoratti, C., et al. Anandamide initiates Ca(2+) signaling via CB2 receptor linked to phospholipase C in calf pulmonary endothelial cells. Br. J. Pharmacol. 2003; 140: 1351–1362.

17. Cabal, G.A. and Griffin-Thomas, l. Emerging Role of the CB2 Cannabinoid Receptor in Immune Regulation and Therapeutic Prospects. Expert Rev. Mol. Med. 2009; 11: e3 doi:10.1017/S1462399409000957.

18. Cabral, G.A., Raborn, E.S., Griffin, L., Dennis,J., Marciano-Cabral, F. CB2 receptors in the brain: role in central immune function. Br. J. Pharmacol. 2008; 153(2): 240–251.

19. Demuth, D.G., Molleman, A. Cannabinoid signaling. Life Sci. 2006; 78:546–563.

20. Bayewitch, M., et al. he peripheral cannabinoid receptor: adenylate cyclase and G protein coupling. FEBS Letter. 1995; 375:143–147.

21. Slipetz, D.M., et al. Activation of the human peripheral cannabinoid receptor results in inhibition of adenylyl cyclase. Mol. Pharmacol. 1995; 48: 352–361.

22. Bouaboula, M., et al. Signaling pathway associated with stimulation of CB2 peripheral cannabinoid receptor. Involvement of both mitogen-activated protein kinase and induction of Krox-24 expression. Eur. J. Biochem. 1996; 237:704–711.

23. Howlett, A.C., Mukhopadhyay, S. Cellular signal transduction by anandamide and 2-arachidonoylglycerol. Chem. Phys. Lipids. 2000; 108: 53–70.

24. Friedman, H., et al. Immuniosupression by marijuana components. In: Alder, R., Felten, D.L., Cohen, N. editors. Psychoneuroimmuniology. Academic Press; 1991.m pp.931–953.

25. Klein, T. et al. Marijuana,immunity and infection. J. Neuroimmunol. 1998; 83: 102–115.

26. Kaminski, N., et al. Suppression of the humoral immune response by cannabinoids is partially mediated through inhibition of adenylate cyclase by a pertussis toxin-sensitive G-protein coupled mechanism. Biochem. Pharmcol. 1994; 48: 1899–1908.

27. Derocq, J., et al. Cannabinoids enhance human B-cell growth at low nanomolar concentrations. FEBS Lett. 1995; 369:177–182.

28. Cabral, G.A., Staab, A. Effects on the immune system. Handb Exp Pharmacol. 2005; 168: 385–423.

29. Morahan, P.S., et al. Effects of cannabinoids on host resistance to Listeria monocytogenes and herpes simplex virus. Infect. Immun. 1979; 23:670–674.

30. Juel-Jensen, B.E. Cannabis and recurrent herpes simplex. Br. Med. J. 1972:4–296

31. Cabral, G.A., Dove-Pettit, D.A. Drugs and immunity: cannabinoids and their role in decreased resistance to infectious diseases. J. Neuroimmunol. 998; 83: 116–123.

32. Klein, T.W., Newton, C., Friedman, H. Cannabinoid receptors and immunity. Immunol Today. 1998; 19: 373–381.

33. Arata,S., et al. Enhanced growth of Legionella pneumophilia in tetrahydrocannabinol-treated macrophages. Proc. Soc. Expp. Biol. Med. 1992; 199: 65–67.

34. Arata, S., et al. Tetrahydrocannabinol treatment suppresses growth restriction of Legionella pneumophilia in murine macrophage cultures. Life Sci. 1991; 49:473–479.

35. Marciano-Cadral, F., et al. Dlta-9-tetrahydrocannabunol (THC), the major psychoactive component of marijuana, exacerbates brain infection by Acanthoamoeba. J. Eukaryot. Microbiol. Supp. 2001:4S-5S.

36. Newton, C.A., Klein, T., Friedman, H. Secondary immunity to Legionella pneumophilia and TH1 activity are suppressed by delta-9-tetrahydrocannabinol injection. Infect. Immun. 1994; 62:4015–4020.

37. Burnette-Curley, D. Cabral, G.A. Differential inhibition of RAW264.7macrophage tumoricidal activity by delta 9-tetrahydrocannabinol. Proc. Soc. Exp. Biol. Med. 1995; 210: 64–76.

38. Coffey, R.G., et al. Tetrahydrocannabinol inhibition of macrophage nitric oxide production. Biochem. Pharmacol. 1996; 52:743–751.

39. Klein, T.W., et al. Marijuana components suppress induction and cytolytic function of murine cytotoxic T cells in vitro and in vivo. J. Toxicol. Environ. Health. 1991; 32:465–477.

40. McCoy, K.L., et al. Cannabinoid inhibition of the processing of intact lysozyme by macrophages: evidence for CB2 receptor participation. L. Pharmacol Exp. Ther. 1999; 289:1620–1625.

41. Raborn, E.S., et al. The Cannabinoid delta-9-tetrahydrocannabinol Mediates Inhibition of Macrophage Chemotaxis to RANTES/CCL5: Linkage to the CB2 receptor. J. Neuroimmune Pharmacol. 2008; 3: 117–129.

42. Sacerdote, P., et al. In vivo and in vitro treatment with synthetic cannabinoid CP55,940 decreases the in vitro migration of macrophages in the rat: involvement of both CB1 and CB2 receptors. J. Neuroimmunol. 2000; 109: 155–163.

43. Massi,P., et al. Relative involvement of cannabinoid 1 and CB2 receptors in the

Delta(9)-tetrahydrocannabinol-induced inhibition of natural killer activity. Eur. J. Pharmacol. 2003; 387: 343–347.

44. Klein, T.W., et al. Delta-9-tetrahydrocannabinol treatment suppresses immunity and early IFN-gamma, IL-12, and IL-12 receptor beta 2 responses to Legionella pneumophilia infection. J. Immunol. 2000; 164: 6461–6466.

45. Zhu, L.X., et al. Delta-9-tetrahydrocannabinol inhibits antitumor immunity by a CB2 receptor-mediated,cytokine-dependent pathway. J. Immunol. 2000; 165: 373–380.

46. Berdyshev, E.V., et al. Influence of fatty acid ethanolamides and delta-9-tetrahydrocannabinol on cytokine and arachidonate release by mononuclear cells. Eur. J. Pharmacol. 1997; 330:1231–240.

47. Joseph, J., et al. Anandamide is an endogenous inhibitor for the migration of tumor cells and T lymphocytes. Cancer Immunol. Immunother. 2004; 53:723–728.

48. Valk, P., et al. Anandamide, a natural ligand for the peripheral cannabinoid receptor is a novel synergistic growth factor for hematopoietic cells. Blood. 1997; 90: 1448–1457.

49. Jorda, M.A., et al. Hematopoietic cells expressing the peripheral cannabinoid receptor migrate in rsponsr to the endocannabinoid 2-arachadonylglycerol. Blood. 2002:99:2786–2793.

50. Rayman, N., Lam, K.H., Laman, J.D., Simons,P.J., Lowenberg, B., Sonneveld, P., Delwel, R. Distinct expression profiles of the peripheral cannabinoid receptor in lymphoid tissues depending on receptor activation status. J. Immunol. 2004; 172:2111–2117.

51. Klein, T.W., Friedman,H. Modulation of murine immune cell function by marijuana components. In: Watson, R. editor. Drugs of Abuse and Immune Function. CRC Press; 1990.pp87–111.

52. Burnette-Curley, D., et al. Delta-9-tetrahydrocannabinol inhibits cell contact-dependent cytotoxicity of Bacillus Calmette-Guerin-activated macrophages. Int. J. Immunopharmacol. 1993; 15: 371–382.

53. Cabral, G.A., Mishkin, E.M. Delta-9-tetrahydrocannabinol inhibits macrophage protein expression in response to bacterial immunomodulation. J. Toxicol. Environ. Health. 1989; 26:175–182.

54. Watzl, B., et al. Influences of marijuana components (thc and CBD) on human mononuclear cell cytokine secretion in vitro. In: Freidman, H., Spectur,S., Klein, T.W., editors. Advances in Experimental Medicine and Biology. Plenum Press; 1991. Pp. 63–70.

55. Nakano,Y., et al. Modulation of interleukin 2 activity by delta-9-tertrhydrocannabinol after stimulation with concanavalin A, phytohemagglutinin, or anti-CD3 antibody. Proc. Soc.Exp. Biol. Med. 1992; 201:165–168.

56. Puffenbarger, R.A., et al. Cannabinoids inhibit LPS-inducible cytokine mRNA expression in rat microglial cells. Glia. 2000; 29: 58–69.

57. Jeon, Y.L., et al. Attenuation of inducible nitric oxide gene expressin by delta-9-tetrahydrocannabinol is mediated through the inhibition of nuclear factor-xB/Rel activation. Mol. Pharmacol. 1996; 50:334–341.

58. Adams, D.O., Hamilton, T. A. The cell biology of macrophage activation. Annu. Rev. Immunol. 1984; 2: 283–318.

59. Hamilton T.A., Adams, D.O. Molecular mechanisms of signal transduction in macrophages. Immunol. Today. 1987; 8:151–158.

60. Hamilton, T. A., et al. Effects of bacterial lipopolysaccharide on protein synthesis in murine peritoneal macrophages: Relationship to activation for macrophages tumoricidal function. J Cell Physiol. 1986; 128: 9–17.

61. Carslile, S. et al. Differential expression of the CB2 cannabinoid receptor by rodent macrophages and macrophage like cells in relation to cell activation. Int. Immunopharmacol. 2002; 2: 69–82.

62. Kaplan, B.L.F., Springs, A.E.B., Kaminski, N.E. The Profile of Immune Modulation by Cannabidiol (CBD) Involves Deregulation of Nuclear Factor of Activated T Cells (NFAT). Biochem. Pharmacol. 2008; 76(6): 726–737 doi: 10.1016/j.bcp.2008.06,022.

63. Seivastava, M.D., Srivastava, B.I., Brouhard, B. Delta-9-tetrahydrocannabinol and

cannabidiol altercytokine production by human immune cells. Immunopharmacollogy. 1998; 40(3):179–85.

64. Schuh, K., Twardzik, T., Kneitz, B., Heyer, J., Schimpl, A., Serfling, E. The interleukin 2 receptor alpha chain/ CD 25 promotor is a target for nuclear factor of activated T Cells. J. Exp. Med. 1998; 188(7):1367–73.

65. Harris, H. Chemotaxis of monocytes. Br. J. Exp. Pathol. 1953; 34:276–279.

66. Harris, H. Role of chemotaxis in inflammation. Physiol. Rev. 1954; 34:529–562.

67. Jin, J., Hereld, D. Moving toward understanding eukaryotic chemotaxis. Eur. J. Cell Biol. 2006; 85:905–913.

68. Kehrl,J.H. Chemoattractant receptor signaling and the control of lymphocyte migration. Immunol. Res. 2006; 34:211–227.

69. Becker, E.L. Stimulated neutrophil locomotion: chemokinesis and chemotaxis. Arch. Pathol.Lab Med. 1977; 101:509–513.

70. Keller, H.U., et al. Distinct chemokinetic and chemotactic responses in neutrophil granulocytes. Eur. J. Immunol. 1978; 8:1–7.

71. Lauffenburger, D.A., Horwitz, A.F. Cell migration: A physically integrated molecular process. Cell. 1996; 84: 359–369.

72. Mitchison, T.J., Cramer, L.P. Actin-based cell motility and cell locomotion. Cell. ˋ1996; 84: 371–379.

73. Murdoch, C., Finn, A. Chemokine receptor and their role in inflammation and infectious disease. Blood. 2000; 95:3032–3043.

74. Schiffmann, E., et al. N-formyl-mrtionyl peptides as chemoattractants for leucocytes. Proc. Natl. Acad. Sci. USA. 1975; 72:1059–1062.

75. Gildman, D.W., Goetzel, E.J. Specific binding of leukotriene B4 to receptors on human polymorphonuclear leukocytes. J. Immunol. 1982; 129:1600–1604.

76. Hanahan, D.J. Platelet activating factor: A biologically active phosphoglyceride. Annu. Rev. Biochem. 1986; 55: 483–509.

77. Gerard, C., Gerard, N.P. C5a anaphylatoxin and its seven transmembrane-segment receptor. Annu. Rev. Immunol. 1994; 12:775–808.

78. Baggiolini, M., et al. Interleukin-8 and related chemotactic cytokines CXC and CC chemokines. Adv. Immunol. 1994; 55: 97–179.

79. Baggiolini, M., et al. Human chemokines: an update. Annu. Rev. Immunol. 1997; 15: 675–705.

80. Kim, C.H. Chemokine-chemokine receptor network in immune cell trafficking. Curr. Drug Targets Immune Endocr. Metabol. Disord. 2004; 4:343–361.

81. Le, Y., et al. Chemokines and chemokine receptors: their manifold roles in homeostasis and disease. Cell Mol. Immunol. 2004; 1:95–104.

82. Charo, I.F., Ransohoff,R.M. Mechanisms of disease: The many roles of chemokines and chemokine receptors in inflammation. N. Engl. J. Med. 2006; 354:610–621.

83. Sacerdote, P., et al. The nonpsychoactive component of marijuana cannabidiol modulates chemotaxis and IL-10 and IL-12 production of murine macrophages both in vivo and in vitro .J. Neuroimmunol. 2005; 159: 97–105.

84. Walter, L., et al. Nonpsychotrophic cannabinoid receptors regulate microglial cell migration. J. Neurosci. 2003; 23:1398–1405.

85. Booz,G.W. Cannabidiol as an emergent therapeutic strategy for lessening the impact of inflammation on oxidative stress. Free Radical Biol.& Med. 2011; 51: 1054–1061.

86. Pertwee,R. G., The diverse CB1 and CB2 receptor pharmacology of three plant cannabinoids: delta-9-tetrahydrocannabinol, cannabidiol and delta-9-tetrahydrocannbivarin. Br. J. Pharmacol. 2008; 153: 199–215.

87. Walter, L., Franklin,A., Witting,A., Wade,C., Xie,Y., Kunos,G., Mackie, K., Stella, N. Nonpsychortrophic cannabinoid receptors regulate microglial cell migration. J. Neurosci. 2013; 23: 1398–1405.

88. Ignatowska-Jankowski,B., Jankowski, M., Glac,W., Swiergel,A. H., Cannabidiol-induced lymphopenia does not involve NKT and NK cells.J. Physiol. Pharmacol. 2009; 60(3): 99–103.

SEIZURES

1. Cabral, G. A., Griffin-Thomas, L. Emerging role of the CB2 cannabinoid receptor in

immune regulation and Therapeutic prospects. Expert Rev. Mol. Med. 2009; 11: e3. Doi:10.1017/S1462399409000957.

2. Carlisle, S., et al. Differential expression of the CB2 cannabinoid receptor by rodent macrophages and macrophage-like cells in relation to cell activqtion. Int. Immunopharmacol. 2002; 69: 69–82.

3. Waksman, Y., et al. The central cannabinoid receptor (CB1) mediates inhibition of nitric oxide production by rat microglial cells. J. Pharmacol. Exp. Ther. 1999; 288: 1357–1366.

4. Carrier, E. J., et al. Cultured rat microglial cells synthesize the endocannabinoid 2-arachidonylglycerol, which increases proliferation via a CB2 receptor-dependent mechanism. Mol. Pharmacol. 2004; 65: 999–1007.

5. Walter, L., et al. Nonpsychotropic cannacinoid receptors regulate microglial cell migration. J. Neurosci. 2003; 23: 1398–1405.

6. Fernandez-Ruiz, J., et al. Cannabinoid CB2 receptor: a new target for controlling neural cell survival? Trends Pharmacol. Sci. 2007; 28:39–45.

7. Yiangou, Y., et al. Cox-2, CB2 and P2X7-immunioreactivities are increased in activated microglial cells/ macrophages of multiple sclerosis and amyotrophic lateral sclerosis spinal cord. BMC Neurol. 2006; 6:12.

8. Benito, C., et al. A glial endogenous cannabinoid system is upregulated in the brains of macaques with simian immunodeficiency virus-induced encephalitis. J. Neurosci. 2005; 25: 2530–2536.

9. Zhang, J., et al. Induction of CB2 receptors in the rat spinal cord of neuropathic but not inflammatory chronic pain models. Eur. J. Neurosci. 2003; 17: 2750–2754.

10. Benito, C., et al. Cannabinoid CB1 and CB2 receptors and fatty acid amide hydrolase are specific markers of plaque cell subtypes in human multiple sclerosis. J. Neurosci. 2007; 27: 2396–2402.

11. Maresz,K., e al. Modulation of the cannabinoid CB2 receptor in microglial cells in response to inflammatory stimuli. J. Neurochem. 2005; 95: 437–445.

12. Ashton, J. C., et al. Cerebral hypoxia-ischemic and middle cerebral artery occlusion induce expression of the cannabinoid CB2 receptor in the brain. Neurosci. Lett. 2007; 412: 114–117.

13. Benito, C., et al Cannabinoid CB2 receptors and fatty acid amide hydrolase are selectively overexpressed in neuritic plaque-associated glia in Alzheimer's disease brains. J. Neurosci. 2003; 23: 11136–11141.

14. Carrier, E. J., et al. Endocannabinoids in neuroimmunology and stress. Curr. Drug Targets CNS Neurol Discord. 2005; 4: 657–665.

15. Sacerdote, P., et al. The nonpsychotrophic component of marijuana cannabidiol modulates chemotaxis and IL-10 and IL-12 production of murine macrophage both in vivo and in vitro. J. Neuroimmunol. 2005; 159:97–105.

16. Harris, H. Role of chemotaxis in inflammation. Physiol Rev. 1954; 34:529–562.

17. McCoy, K.L., et al. Cannabinoid inhibition of the processing of intact lysozyme by macrophages: evidence for CB2 receptor participation. J. Pharmacol. Exp. Ther. 1999; 289: 1620–1625.

18. Buckley, N, E., et al. Immunomodulation by cannabinoids id absent in mice deficient for the cannabinoid CB(2) receptor. Eur. J. Pharmacol. 2000; 396:141–149.

19. Carlisle, S., et al. Differential expression of the CB2 cannabinoid receptor by rodent macrophages and macrophage-like cells in relation to cell activation. Int. Immunopharmacol. 2002; 2:69–82.

20. Nunez,E., et al. Cannabinoid CB2 receptors are expressed by perivascular microglial cells in the human brain: an immunohistochemical study. Synapse. 2004; 53: 208–213.

21. Ramirex, B.G., et al. Prevention of Alzheimer's disease pathology by cannabinoids: neuroprotection mediated by blockade of microglial activation. J. Neurosci. 2005; 25: 1904–1913.

22. Cabral, G.A., Marciano-Cabral, F. Cannabinoid receptors in microglia of the central nervous system: immune functional relevance. J. Leukoc. Biol. 2005; 78: 1192–1197.

23. Shohami, E., et al. Cytokine production in the brain following closed head injury: dexanabinol (HU-211) is a novel TNF-alpha inhibitor and an effective neuroprotectant. J. Neuroimmunol. 1997; 72:169–177.

24. Cabral, G. A., et al. Cannabinoid-mediated inhibition of inducible nitric oxide production by rat microglial cells: evidence for CB1 receptor participation. Adv. Exp. Mwd. Biol. 2001; 493: 207–214.

25. Molina-Holdado, F., et al. Role of CB1 and CB2 receptors in the inhibitory effects of cannabinoids on lipopolysaccharide-induced nitric oxide release in astrocyte cultures. J. Neurosci. Res. 2002; 67: 829–36.

26. Klegeris, A., et al. Reduction of human monocytic cell neurotoxicity and cytokine secretion by ligands of the cannabinoid-type CB2 receptor. Br. J. Pharmacol. 2003; 139: 775–786.

27. Sheng, W.S., et al. Synthetic cannabinoid WIN55,212–2 inhibits generation of inflammatory mediators by IK-1beta-stimulated human astrocytes. Glia. 2005; 49: 211–219.

28. Kreutzberg, G.W. Microglia: a sensor for pathological events in the CNS. Trends Neurosci. '1996; 19:312–18.

29. Benveniste, E.N. Role of macrophafges/microglia in multiple sclerosis and experimental allergic encephalomyelitis. J. Mol. Med. 1997; 75: 165–173.

30. Benito,C., Tolon, R.M., Pazos, M.R., Nunez, E., Castillo, A.L., Romero,J. Cannabinoid CB2 receptors in human brain inflammation. Br. J. Pharmacol. 2008; 153(2): 277–285 doi: 10.1038/sj.bip.0707505.

31. Fernandez-Ruis, J.J., Gonzalez, S., Romero, J., Ramos, J.A. Cannabinoids in neurodegeneration and neuroprotection Cannabinoids as Therapeutics 2005. Birkhauser Verlag: Switzerland; 79–109. In: Mechoulam, R. (ed)

32. Grundy, R.I., Rabuffeti, M., Beltramo, M. Cannabinoids and neuroprotection. Mol Neurobio. 2001; 24:29–52.

33. Mechoulam, R., Panikashivili, A., Shohami, E. Cannabinoids and brain injury: therapeutic implications. Trends Mol. Med. 2002; 8: 58–61.

34. Grundy, R.I.. The therapeutic potential of the cannabinoids in neuroprotection. Expert Opin. Investig. Drugs. 2002; 11: 1–10.

35. Guzman,M., Sanchez,C. Effects of cannabinoids on energy metabolism. Life Sci. 1999; 65:657–664.

36. Witting, A., Stella, N. Cannabinoid signaling in glial cells in health and disease. Curr. Neuropharmacol. 2004; 2(1): 115–124.

37. Doble,A. The role of excitotoxicity in neurodegenerative disease: implications for therapy. Pharmacol. Ther. 1999; 81: 163–221.

38. van der Stelt,M., Veldhuis, W.B., Maccarrone,M., Bar, P.R., Nicolay, K. Veldink,G.A., Marzo, V., Vliegenhart, J.F. Acute neuronal injury, excitotoxicity, and the endocannabinoid system. Mol. Neurobiol. 2002; 26: 317–346.

39. Romero, J., Lastres-Becker, I., de Miguel, R., Berrendero, F., Ramos, J. A., Fernandez-Ruis, J.J. The endogenous cannabinoid system and the basal ganglia: biochemical, pharmalogical and therapeutic aspects. Pharmacol. Ther. 2002; 95: 137–152.

40. Shen,M., Thayer, S.A. Cannabinoid receptor agonist protect cultured rat hippocampal neurons from excitotoxicity. Mol. Pharmacol. 1998; 54: 459–462.

41. Abood, M.E., Rizvi,,G., Sallapudi, N., McAllister, S.D. Activation of the CB1 cannabinoid receptor protects cultured mouse spinal neurons against excitotoxicity. Neurosci. Lett. 2001; 309: 197–201,

42. Nagayama, T., Sinor, A.D., Simon, R.P., Chen, J., Graham, S.H., Jin, K.L., Greenberg, D.A. Cannabinoids and neuroprotection in global and focal cerebral ischemia and in neuronal cultures. J. Neurosci. 1999; 19: 2987–2995.

43. Schlicker,E., Kathmann, M. Modulation of transmitter release via presynaptic cannabinoid receptors. Trends Pharmacol. 2001; 22: 565–572.

44. Marsicano, G., Goodenough, S., Monory,K., Hermann, H., Eder, M., Cannich, A., Azad,S.C., Cascio, M.G., Guiterrez, S.O., van

der Stelt, M. CB1 cannabinoid receptors and on-demand ddefense against excitotoxicity. Science. 2003; 302: 84–88.

45. Battaglia, G., Bruno, V., Pisani, A., Centonze,D., Catania, M.V., Calabresi, P., Nicoletti, F. Selective blockade of typr-1 metabotropic glutamate receptors induces neuroprotection by enhancing gabaergic transmission. Mol. Cell Neurosci. 2001; 17:1071–1083.

46. Maneuf,Y.P., Nash, J.E., Croosman,A.R., Brotchie, J.M. Activation of the cannabinoid receptor by D9-THC reduces GABA uptake in the globus pallidus. Eur. J. Pharmacol. 1996; 308: 161–164.

47. Romero, J., de Miguel, R., Ramos, J.A., Fernandez-Ruis, J.J. The activation of cannabinoid receptors in straitonigal neurons inhibited GABA uptake. Life Sci. 1998; 62: 351–363.

48. Saji, M., Blau, A.D., Volpe, B.T. Prevention of transneuronal degeneration of neurons in the substantia nigra reticulate by ablation of the subthalamic nucleus. Exp. Neurol. 1996; 141: 120–129.

49. Fowler, C.J. Plant-derived, synthetic and endogenous cannabinoids as neuroprotective agents. Non-psycho active cannabinoids, 'entourage' compounds and inhibitors of N-acyl-ethanolamine breakdown as therapeutic strategies to avoid psychotropic effects. Brain Res. Rev. 2003; 41: 26–43.

50. Mackie,K., Hille, B. Cannabinoids inhibit N-type calcium channels in neuroblastoma-glioma cells. Proc. Natl. Acad. Sci. USA 1992; 89:3825–3829.

51. Mackie, K., Lai,Y., Westenbrock,R., Mitchell,R. Cannabinoids activate an inwardly rectifying potassium conductance and inhibit Q-type cacium currents in AtT20 cells transfected with rat brain cannabinoid receptors. J. Neurosci. 1995; 15: 6552–6561.

52. Pan,X., Ikeda, S.R., Lewis, D.L. Rat brain cannabinoid receptor modulates N-type Ca2+ channels in a neuronal expression system. Mol. Pharmacol. 1996; 49: 707–714.

53. Gebremedhin, D., Lange, A.R., Campbell, W.B., Hillard, C.J., Harder, D.R. Cannabinoid CB1 receptor of cat cerebral arterial muscle functions to inhibit L-type Ca2+ channel

current. Am. J. Physiol. Heart Circ. Physiol. 1999; 276: H2085-H2093.

54. Chemin,J., Monteil, A., Perez-Reves, E., Nargeot, J., Lory, P. Direct inhibition of T-type calcium channels by the rndogenous cannabinoid anandamide. EMBO J. 2001; 20:7033–7040.

55. Deadwyler, S.A., Hampson, R.E., Bennett, B.A., Edwards, T.A., Mu, J., Pacheco, M.A., Childers, S.R. Cannabinoids modulate potassium current in cultured hippocampal neurons. Recept. Channel. 1993; 1:121–134.

56. McAllister, S.D., Grifin, G., Satin, L.S., Abood, M.E. Cannabinoid receptors can activate and inhibit G protein-coupled inward rectifying potassium channels in a xenopus oocyte expression system. J. Pharmacol. Exp. Ther. 1999; 291: 618–626.

57. Pong, K. Oxidative stress in neurodegenerative diseases: therapeutic implications for super-oxide dismutase mimetics. Expert Opin. Biol. Ther. 2003; 3:127–139.

58. Klein, J.A., Ackerman, S.L. Oxidative stress, cell cycle, and neurodegeneration. J. Clin. Invest. 2003; 111: 785–793.

59. Chan, P.H. Reactive oxygen radicals in signaling and damage in the ischemic brain. J. Cereb. Blood Flow Metab. 2001; 21: 2–14.

60. Marsicano, G., Moorsmann, B., Hermann, H., Lutz,B., Behl, C, Neuroprotective properties of cannabinoids against oxidative stress: role of the cannabinoid receptor CB1. J. Neurochem. 2002; 80: 448–456.

61. Belayev, L., Bar-Joseph, A., Adamchik, J., Biegon, A. HU-211, a nonpsycotrophic cannabinoid improves neurological signs and reduces brain damage after severe forebrain ischemia in rats. Mol. Chem Neuropathol. 1995; 25: 19–33.

62. Braida, D., Pegorini, S., Arcidiacono,M.V., Consalez, G.G., Croci,L., Sala, M. Post-ischemic treatment with cannabidiol prevents electroencephalographic, hyperlocomotion and neuronal injury in gerbils. Neurosci. Lett. 2003; 346: 61–64.

63. Hampson,A.J., Grimaldi, M., Axelrod, J., Wink,D. Cannabidiol and (-)D9-tetrahydrocannabinol are neuroprotective antioxidants Proc. Natl. Acad. Sci. USA. 1998; 95:8268–8273.

64. Malfait, A.M., Galluly, R., Sumariwalla, P.F., Malik, A.S., Andreakos, E., Mechoulam, R., Feldmann, M. The nonpsychoactive cannabis constituent cannabidiol is an oral anti-arthritic therapeutic in murine collagen-induced arthritis. Proc. Natl. Acad. Sci. USA 2000; 97: 9561-9566.

65. Adams, I.B., Martin, B.R. Cannabis: pharmacology and toxicology in animals and humans. Addiction. 1996; 91:1585-1614.

66. Bisogno, T., Hanus, L., DePetrocellis, L., Tchilibon, S., Ponde,D.E., Brandi, I., Moriello, A.S., Davis, J.B., Mechoulam, R., DiMarzo, V. Molecular targets for cannabidiol and its synthetic analogues: effects on vanilloid VR1 receptors and on the cellular uptake and enzymatic hydrolysis of anandamide. Brit. J. Pharmacol. 2001; 134: 845-852.

67. Mechoulam, R., Parker, L.A., Gallily,R. Cannabidiol: an overview of some pharmacological aspects. J. Clin. Pharmacol. 2002; 42: 11S-19S.

68. Liu,B., Hong, J.S. Role of microglia in inflammation-mediated neurodegenerative diseases: mechanisms and strategies for therapeutic interventions. J. Pharmacol. Exp. Ther. 2003; 304: 1-7.

69. Walter, L., Stella, N. Cannabinoids and neuroinflammation. Br. J. Pharmacol. 2004; 141: 775-785.

70. Aloisi, F. The role of microglia and astrocytes in CNS immune surveillance and immunopathology. Adv. Exp. Med. Biol. 1999; 468: 123-133.

71. Iadecola,C., Alexander,M. Cerebral ischemia and inflammation. Curr. Opin. Neurol. 2001; 14: 89-94.

72. Dusart, I., Schwab, M.E. Secondary cell death and the inflammatory reaction after dorsal hemisection of the rat spinal cord. Eur. J. Neurosci. 1994; 6:712-724.

73. McGeer, P.L., Yasojima, K., McGeer, E.G. Inflammation in Parkinson's disease. Adv Neurol. 2001; 86:·83-89.

74. Sapp, E., Kegel, K.B., Aronin, N., Hashikawa, T., Tohyama, K., Bhide, P.G., Vonsattel, J.P., DiFiglia,M. Early and progressive accumulation of reactive microglia in the Huntington disease brain. J. Neuropathol. Exp. Neurol. 2001; 60: 161-172.

75. McGeer, P.L., Rogers,J. Anti-inflammatory agents as a therapeutic approach to Alzheimer's disease. Neurology. 1992; 42: 447-449.

76. Eikelenboom, P., Bate, C., Van Gool, W.A., Hoozemans, J.J., Rozemuller,J.M., Veerhuis, R., Williams,A. Neuroinflammation in Alzheimers disease and prion disease. Glia. 2002; 40:232-239.

77. Baker, D., Pryce, G. The therapeutic potential of cannabis in multiple sclerosis. Expert Opin. Investing. Drugs. 2003; 12:561-567.

78. Witting,A., Stwella, N. Cannabinoid signaling in glial cells in health and disease. Curr. Neuropharmacol. 2004; 2(1): 115-124.

79. Shohami, E., Mechoulam, R. A non-psychotropic cannabinoid with neuroprotective properties. Drug Dev.Res. 2000; 50:211-215.

80. Waksman,Y., Olson, J.M., Carlisle, S.J., Cabral, G.A. The central cannabinoid receptor (CB1) mediates inhibition of nitric oxide production by rat microglial cells. J. Pharmacol. Exp. Ther. 1999; 288: 1357-1366.

81. Molina-Holgado, F., Lledo, A., Guaza, C. Anandamide suppresses nitric oxide and TNF-alpha responses to Theiler's virus or endotoxin in astrocytes. Neuroreport. 1997; 8: 1929-1933.

82. Hillard,C.J., Muthian, S., Kearn, C.S. Effects of CB(1) cannabinoid receptor activation on cerebellar granule cell nitric oxide synthase activity. FEBS Lett. 1999; 459: 277-281.

83. Coffey, R.G., Snella, E., Johnson K., Pross, S. Inhibition of macrophage nitric oxide production by tetrahydrocannabinol in vivo and in vitro. Int. Immunopharmacol. 1996; 18: 749-752.

84. Smith, S.R., Terminelli, C., Denhardt, G. Effects of cannabinoid receptor agonist and antagonist ligands on production of inflammatory cytokines and anti-inflammatory interleukin-10 in endotoxemic mice. J. Pharmacol. Exp. Ther. 2000; 293: 136-150.

85. Polazzi, E., Gianni,T., Contestabile, A. Microglial cells protect cerebellar granule neurons from apoptosis: evidence for reciprocal signaling. Glia. @001; 36: 271-280.

86. Molina-Holgado, F., Pinteau, E., Moore, J.D., Molina-Holgado, E., Guaza, C.,

Gibson, R.M., Rothwell, N.J. Endogenous interleukin-1 receptor antagonist mediates anti-inflammatory and neuroprotective actions of cannabinoids in neurons and glia. J. Neurosci. 2003; 23: 6470–6474.

87. Benito, C., Nunez, E., Tolon, R.M., Rabano, A., Hillard, C.J., Romero, J. Cannabinoid CB2 receptors and fatty acid amide hydrolase are selectively overexpressed in neuritic plaque-associated glia in Alzheimer's disease brains. J. Neurosci. 2003; 23: 11136–11141.

88. Skaper, S.D., Buriani, A., Dal Toso, R., Petrelli, L., Romanello,S., Facci, L., Leon,A. The ALIAmide palmitoylethanolamide and cannabinoids, but not anandamide, are protective in a delayed postglutamate paradigm of excitotoxic death in cerebellar granule neurons. Proc. Natl. Acad. Sci. USA. 1996; 93: 3984–3989.

89. Sanchez, C., de Ceballos, M.L., del Pulgar, T.G., Rueda, D., Corbacho,C., Velasco,G., Galve-Ropert, I., Huffman, J.W., Ramon y Cajal, S., GuzmaN,M. Inhibition of glioma growth in vivo by selective activation of the CB2 cannabinoid receptor. Cancer Res. 2001; 61: 5784–5789.

90. Nunez, E., Benito,C., Pazos, M.R., Barbachano, A., Fajardo, O., Gonzalez, S., Tolon, R.M., Romero, J. Cannabinoid CB2 receptors are expressed by perivascular microglial cells in the human brain: am immunohistochemical study. Sunapse. 2004; 53: 208–213.

91. Walter,L., Franklin, A., Witting, A., Wade, C., Xie, Y., Kunos,G., Mackie, K., Stella,N. Nonpsychotropic cannabinoid receptors regulate microglial cell migration. J Neurosci. 2003; 23: 1398–1405.

92. Carrier, E.J., Kearn, C.S., Barkmeier, A.J., Breese, N.M., Yang, W., Nithipatikom, K., Pfister, S.L., Campbell, W.B., Hillard, C.J. Cultured rat microglial cells synthesize the endocannabinoid 2-arachidonylglycerol, which increases proliferation via CB2 receptor-dependent mechanism. Mol. Pharmacol. 2004; 65: 999–1007.

93. Giulian, D. Microglial and the immune pathology of Alzheimer's disease. Am. J. Hum. Genet. 1999; 65: 13–18.

94. Rubanyi, G.M., Polokoff, M.A. Endothelins: molecular biology, biochemistry, pharmacology, physiology and pathophysiology. Pharmacol. Rev. 1994; 46: 325–415.

95. Schinelli, S. The brain endothelin system as potential target for brain-related pathologies. Curr. Drug Targets CNS Neurol. Disord. 2002; 1: 543–553.

96. Wagner, J.A., Varga, K., Kunos,G. Cardiovascular actions of cannabinoids and their generation during shock. J. Mol. Med. 1998; 76: 824–836.

97. Randall, M.D., Harris, D., Kendall,D.A., Ralevic,V, Cardiovascular effects of cannabionids. Pharmacol. Ther. 2002; 95: 191–202.

98. Mechoulam, R., Spatz, M., Shohami,E. Endovcannabinoids and neuroprotection. Sci. STKE 129/RES.

99. Chen, Y., McCarron, R.M., Ohara, Y., Bembry,J., Azzam, N., Lenz, F.A., Shohami,E., Mechoulam, R., Spatz, M. Human brain capillary endothelium: 2-arachidonylglycerol (endocannabinoid) interacts with endothelin-1. Circ. Res. 2000; 87: 323–327.

100. Hillard, C.J. Endocannabinoids and vascular function. J. Pharmacol. Exp. Ther. 2000; 294: 27–32.

101. Graham, D.I., McIntosh, T.K., Maxwell,W.L., Nicoll, J.A. Recent advances in neurotrama. J. Neuropathol. Exp. Neurol. 2000; 59:641–651.

102. Janardhan, V., Qureshi, A.I. Mechanisms of ischemic brain injury. Curr Cardiol Rep. 2004; 6: 117–123.

103. Alexi, T., Borlongan, C.V., Faull, R. L., Williams, C.E., Clark, R.G., Gluckman, P.D., Hughs, P.E. Neuroprotective strategies for basal ganglia degeneration: Parkinson's and huntington's disease. Prog. Neurobio. 2000; 60: 409–470.

104. Moosman, B., Behl, C. Antioxidants as treatment for neurodegenerative disorders. Expert. Opin. Invest. Drugs 2002; 11: 1407–1435.

105. Rodnitzky, R.L. Can calcium antagonists provide a neuroprotective effect in Parkinson's disease? Drugs 1999; 57: 845–849.

106. Galea, E., Heneka, M.T., Dello Russo, C., Feinstein, D.L. Intrinsic regulation of brain inflammatory responses. Cell Mol. Neurobio. 2003; 23: 625–635.

107. Gagliadi, R.J. Neuroprotection, excitotoxicity, and NMDA antagonist. Arq. Neuropsiquiatr. 2000; 58:583–588.

108. Marsicano, G., Goodenough, S., Monory, K., Hermann, H., Eder, M., Cannich, A., Azad, S.C., Cascio, M.G., Guitierrez,S.O., van der Stelt, M. et al. CB1 cannabinid receptors and on-demand defense against excitotoxicity. Science. 2003; 302: 84–88.

109. Nagayama, T., Sinor, A.D., Simon, R.P., Chen, J., Graham, S.H., Jin, K.L., Greenberg, D.A. Cannabinoids and neuroprotection in global and focal cerebral ischemia and in neuronal cultures. J. Neurosci. 1999; 19: 2987–2995.

110. Louw, D.F., Yang, F.W., Sutherland, G.R. The effect of D9-tetrahydrocannabinol on forebrain ischemia in rat. Brain Res. 2000; 857: 183–187.

111. Mauler, F., Mittendorf, J., Horvath, E., DeVry, L. Characterization of the diarylether sulfonylester (-)(R)-3-(2-hydroxymethylindanyl-4-oxy)phenyl-4,4,4-trifluoro-1-sulfonate (BAY38–7271) as a potent cannabinoid receptor agonist with neuroprotective properties. J. Pharmacol. Exp. Ther. 2002; 302: 359–368.

112. Sinor, A.D., Irvin, S.M., Greenberg, D.A. Endocannabinoids protect cerebral cortical neurons from in vitro ischemia in rats. Neurosci. Lett. 2000; 278: 157–160.

113. Panikashvili, D., Simeonidou, C., Ben-Shabat, S., Hanus, L., Breuer, A., Mechoulam, R., Shohami, E. An endogenous cannabinoid (2-AG) is neuroprotective after brain injury. Nature. 2001; 413: 527–531.

114. Fernandez-Ruis, J. J., Romero, J., Velasco,G., Tolon, R.M., Ramos, J.A., Guzman, M. Cannabinoid CB2 receptors: a new target for controlling neural cell survival. TRENDS Pharmacol. Sci. 2007; 28(1): 39–45.

115. van der Stelt, M., Veldius, W.B., Maccarrone, M., Bar, P.R., Nicolay, K., Veldink, G.A., DiMarzo, V., Vliegenthart, J. F. Acute neuronal injury, excitotoxicity, and the endocannabinoid system. Mol. Neurobio. 2002; 26: 317–346.

116. Stella,N. Cannabinoid signaling in glial cells. Glia. 2004; 48:267–77.

117. Beltramo, M., Bernardini, N., Bertorelli, R., Campanella, M., Nicolussi, E., Fredduzzi, S., et al. CB2 receptor-mediated antihyperalgesia: possible direct involvement of neural mechanisms. Eur. J. Neurosci. 2006; 23:1530–1538.

118. Mukhopadhyay, S., Das, S., Williams, E.A., Moore, D., Jones, J.D., Zahm, D.S., et al. Lypopolysaccharide and cyclic AMP regulation of CB2 cannabinoid receptor levels in rat brain and mouse RAW 264.7 macrophages. J. Neuroimmunol. 2006; 181: 82–92.

119. Ashton, J.C., Rahman, R.M.A., Nair, S.M., Sutherland, B.A., Glass, M., Appleton, I. Cerebral hypoxia-ischemia and middle cerebral artery occlusion induced expression of the cannabinoid CB2 receptor in the brain. Neurosci. Lett. 2007; 412: 114–117.

120. Palazuelos, J., Aguado, T., Egia, A., Mechoulam,R., Guzman,M., Galve-Roperh, I. Non-psychoactive CB2 cabanoid agonist stimulate neural progenitor proliferation. FASEB J. 2006; 20: 2405–2407.

121. Molina-Holgado,E., Vela, J.M., Arevalo-Martin, A., Almazan,G., Molina-Holgado, F et al. Cannabinoids promote oligodendrocytes progenitor survival: involvement of cannabinoid receptors and phosphatidylinositol-3 kinase.Akt signaling. J. Neurosci. 2002; 22: 9742–9753.

122. Ross, R.A., Coutts, A.A., McFarland, S.M., Anavi-Goffer,S., Irving, A.J., Pertwee, R.G., et al. Actions of cannabinoid receptor ligands on rat cultured sensory neurons: implications for antinocioception. 2001; 40: 221–232.

123. Stander,S., Schmelz,M., Metze, D., Luger,T., Rukwied, R. Distribution of cannabinoid receptor 1 (CB1) and 2 (CB2) on sensory nerve fibers and adnexal structures in human skin. J. Dermatol. Sci. 2005; 38: 177–188.

124. Wotherspoon, G., Fox, A., McIntyre, P., Colley, S., Bevan, S., Winter, J. Peripheral nerve injury induces cannabinoid receptor

2 protein expression in rat sensory neurons. Neurosci. 2005; 135: 235–245.

125. Van Sickle, M.D., Duncan, M., Kingsley, P.J., Mouihate, A., Urbani, P. et al. Identification and functional characterization of brainstem cannabinoid CB2 receptors. 2005; 310: 329–332.

126. Beltramo,M., Bernardini, N., Bertorelli, R., Campanella, M., Nicolussi, E., et al. CB2 receptor-mediated antihyperalgesia: possible direct involvement of neural mechanisms. 2006; 23:1530–1538.

127. Howlett, A,C., Barth, F., Bonner, T.I., Cabral, G., Casellas, P., Devane, W.A., Felder, C.C., Herkenham, M., Mackie, K., Martin, B.R., Mechoulam, R., Pertwee, R.G., International Union of Pharmacology. XXVII. Classification of cannabinoid receptors. Pharmacol. Rev. 2002; 54: 161–202.

128. Bouaboula, M., Pinot-Chazel,C., Marchand, J., Canat, X., Bourrie, B., Rinaldi-Carmona, M., Calandra, B., LeFur, G., Casellas,P. Signaling pathway associated with stimulation of CB2 peripheral cannabinoid receptor. Involvement of both mitogen-activated protein kinase and induction of Krox-24 expression. Eur. J. Biochem. 1996; 237: 704–711.

129. Gertsch, J., Schoop, R., Kuenzle, U., Suter, A. Echinacea alkylamides modulate TNF-alpha gene expression via cannabinoid receptor CB2 and multiple signal transduction pathways. FEBS Lett. 2004; 577: 563–569.

130. Herrera, B., Carracedo, A., Diez-Zaera, M., Guzman, M., Velasco, G. p38 MAPK is involved in CB2 receptor induced apoptosis of human leukemia cells. FEBS Lett. 2005; 579: 5084–5088.

131. Samson, M.T., Small-Howard, A., Shimoda, L.M., Koblan-Huberson, M., Stokes, A.J., Turner, H. Differential roles of CB1 and CB2 cannabinoid receptors in mast cells. J. Immunol. 2003; 170: 4953–4962.

132. Carracedo,A., Lorente, M., Eia, A., Blazquez, C., Garcia, S., Giroux, V., et al. The stress regulated protein p8 mediates cannabinoid-induced apoptosis of tumor cells. Cancer Cell. 2006; 9:301–312.

133. Carracedo, A., Gironella, M., Lorente, M., Garcia, S., Guzman, M., Iovanna, J.L.

Cannabinoids induce apoptosis of pancreatic tumor cells via endoplasmic reticulum stress-related genes. Cancer Res. 2006; 66: 6748–6755.

134. Onaivi, E.S., Ishiguro, H., Gong, J.P. Patel, S., Perchuk, A., Meozzi, P.A., et al. Discovery of the presence and functional expression of cannabinoid CB2 receptors in the brain. Ann. NY Acad. Sci. 2006; 1074: 514–536.

135. Alberich Jorda, M., Rayman, N., Tas, M., Verbakel, S.E., Battista, N., van Lom, K., et al. The peripheral cannabinoid receptor CB2, frequently expressed on AML blasts, either induces a neutrophilic differentiation block or confers abnormal migration properties in a ligand-dependent manner. Blood 2004; 104: 526–534.

136. van der Stelt, M., DiMarzo, V. Cannabinoid receptors and their role in neuroprotection. Neuromolecular Med. 2005; 7: 37–50.

137. Piomwlli, D. The molecular logic of endocannabinoid signaling. Nat. Rev. Neurosci. 2003; 4: 873–878.

138. Mackie, K. Cannabinoid receptors as therapeutic targets. Annu. Rev. Pharmacol. Toxicol. 2006; 46: 101–122.

139. Guzman, M., Sanchez, C., Galve-Roperh, I. Cannabinoids and cell fate. Pharmacol. Ther. 2002; 95(2): 175–184.

140. Guzman, M. Cannabinoids: potential anticancer agents. Natl. Rev. Cancer 2003; 3:745–755.

141. Caffarel, M.M. et al. Delta-9-tetrahydrocannabinol inhibits human breast cancer cell cycle by down-regulating Cdc2. Cancer Res. 2006; 66: 6615–6621.

142. Mechoulam, R., Panikashvili, D., Shohami, E. Cannabinoids and brain injury: therapeutic implications. Trends Mol. Med. 2002; 8(2): 58–61.

143. Eljaschewitsch, E.,et al. The endocannabinoid anandamide protects neurons during CNS inflammation by induction of MKP-1 in microglial cells. Neuron. 2006; 49: 67–79.

NEUROPROTECTION

1. Skaper, S.D., Buriani, A., Dal Toso, R., Petrelli, L., Romanello, S., Facci,L., et al. The ALIAmide

palmitoyethanolamide and cannabinoids, but not anandamide, are protectivr in a delayed postglutamate paradigm of excitotoxic death in cerebellar graniule neurons. Proc. Natl Acad Sci USA 1996; 93:3984–9

2. Shen, M., Thayer, S.A. Cannabinoid receptor agonists protect cultured rat hippocampal neurons fron excitotoxicity Mol Pharmacol 1998; 54:459–62

3. Nagayama, T., Sinor, A.D., Simon, R.R., Chen, J., Graham, S.H., Jin, K., et al. Cannabinoids and neuroprotection in global and focal cerebral ischemia and in neuronal cultures. J. Neurosci 1999; 19:2987–95.

4. Galve-Roperh, I., Aguado, T., Palazuelos, J., Guzman, M. Mechanisms of Control of Neuron Survival by the Endocannabinoid System. Cur Pharmaceutical Design 2008; 14(23):2279–88.

5. Freund, T.F., Katona, I., Piomelli, D. Role of Endogenpous Cannabinoids in synaptic signaling. Physiol Rev2003; 83:1017–66

6. Chevaleyre, V., Takahashi, K.A., Castillo, P.E. Endocannabinoid-mediated synaptic plasticity in the CNS. Ann Rev Neurosci 2006; 29:37–76

ALZHEIMER'S DISEASE

1. Fernandez-Ruis, J.J., Gonzalez, S., Romero, J., Ramos, J.A. Cannabinoids in neurodegeneration and neuroprotection. Cannabinoids as Therapeutics. 2005. Birkhauser Verlag: Switzerland; 79–109. In: Mechoulam, R. (ed)

2. Fernandez-Ruis, J., de Miguel, R., Hernandez,M., Cebeira, M., Ramos, J.A. Endocannabinoids and Dopamine-Related Functions in the CNS. Endocannabinoids The Brain and Body's Marijuana and Beyond. 2006 CRC Press, Boca Raton, Fla. 261–290. In: Onaivi,E., Sugiura,T., DiMarzo,V. (ed)

3. Fernandez-Ruis,J., Romero,J., Velasco, G., Tolon,R.M., Ramos, J.A., Guzman, M. Cannabinoid CB2 receptor: a new target for controlling neural cell survival? Trends Pharmacol. Sci. 2007; 28(1): 39–45.

4. Esposito, G., Scuderi, C., Valenza, M., Togna, G.I., Latina, V., et al. Cannabidiol reduces ABeta- induced neuroinflammation and promotes hippocampal neurogenesis through PPAR-gamma involvement. PLoS ONE 6: e28668. Doi: 10.1371/jornal.pone.0028668.

5. Campbell, V.A., Gowran, A. Alzheimer's disease; taking the edge off with cannabinoids? Br. J. Pharmacol. 2007; 152(5): 655–662.

6. Aso, E., Ferrer, I. Cannabinoids for the treatment of Alzheimer's disease: moving toward the clinic. Front. Pharmacol. 2014. Doi: 10.33891/fphar.2014.00037.

7. Herbert, L.E., Scherr, P.A., Bienias, J.L., Bennett, D.A., Evans, D.A. Alzheimer's disease in the US population: Prevalence estimates using the 2000 census. Archiv. Neurol. 2003:60: 1119–1122.

8. Walsh, D.M., Selkoe, D.L. Beta-amyloid oligomers-a decade of discovery. J. Neurochem. 2007; 101: 1172–1184.

9. Boland, B., Campbell, V. Amyloid-induced apoptosis of cultured cortical neurons involves calpain-mediated cleavage of poly-ADP ribose polymerase. Neurobio. Aging. 2003; 24: 179–186.

10. Ogomori, K., Kitamoto, T., Tateishi, J., Sato, Y., Suetsugu, M., Abe, M. Protein amyloid is widely distributed in the central nervous system of patients with Alzheimer's disease. Am. aJ. Pathol. 1989; 134: 243–251.

11. Mi, K., Johnson, G.V., The role of tau phosphorylation in the pathogenesis of Alzeheimer's disease. Curr. Alzheimer Res. 2006; 3: 449–463

12. Rich, J.B., Rasmusson, D.X., Folstein, M.F., Carson, K.A., Kawas, C., Brandt, J. Nonsteroidal anti-inflammatory drugs in Alzheimer's disease. Neurology. 1995; 45:51–55.

13. Wilkinson, B.L., Landreth, G.E. The microglial NADPH oxidase complex as a source of oxidative stress in Alzheimer's disease. J. Neuroinflam. 2006; 3: 30–42.

14. Bayer, T.A., Buslei, R., Havas, L., Falkai, P. Evidence for activation of microglia in patients with psychiatric illnesses. Neurosci. Lett. 1999; 271: 126–128.

15. Heneka, M.T., O'Banion, M.K. Inflammotory processes in Alzheimer's disease. J. Neuroimmunol. 2007; 184: 69–91.

16. Vereker,E., Campbell, V., Roche, E., McEntee, E., Lynch, M.A. Lipopolysaccharide inhibits

long-term potentiation in the rat dentate gyrus by activation of caspase-1. J. Biol. Chem. 2000; 275: 26252–26258.

17. LaFerla, F.M. Calcium dyshomeostasis and intracellular signaling in Alzheimer's disease. Nat. Rev. Neurosci. 2002; 3: 862–872.

18. Volicer, L., Stelly, M., Morris, J., McLaughlin, J., Volicer, B.J. Effects of Dronabinol on anorexia and disturbed behavior in patients with Alzheimer's disease. Int. J. Geriatr. Psych. 1997; 12: 913–919.

19. Walther, S., Mahlberg, R., Eichman, U., Kunz, D. Delta-9-Tetrahydrocannabinol for nighttime agitation in severe dementia. Psychopharmacology. 2006; 185: 524–528.

20. Jackson, S.J., Diemel, L.T., Pryce, G., Baker, D. Cannabinoids and neuroprotection in CNS inflammatory diseas. J. Neurol. Sci. 2005; 233: 21–25.

21. Herkenham, M., Lynn, A.B., Johnson, M.R., Melvin, L.S., de Costa, B.R., Rice, K.C. Characterization and localization of cannabinoid receptors in rat brain; A Quantitative in vitro autoradiographic study. J. Neurosci. 1991; 11: 563–583.

22. Riedel, G., Davis, S.N. Cannabinoid function in learning, memory and plasticity. Han.db Exp. Pharmacol. 2005; 168: 445–477.

23. Van Sickle, M.C., Duncan, M., Kingsley, P.J., Mouihate, A., Urbani, P., Mackie, K. et al. Identification and functional characterization of brainstem cannabinoid CB2 receptors. Science. 2005; 310: M329–332.

24. Ashton, J.C., Friberg, D., Darlington, C.L., Smith, P.F. Expression of the cannabinoid CB2 receptorr in the rat cerebellum: an immuniohistochemical study. Neurosci. Lett. 2006; 396: 113–116.

25. Nunez, E., Benito, C., Pazos, M.R., Barbachano,A., Fajardo,O., Gonzalez, S. et al. Cannabinoid CB2 receptors are expressed by perivascular microglial cells in the human brain: an immuniohistochemical study. Synapse. 2004; 53: 208–213.

26. Ramirez, B.G., Blazquez, C., Gomez del Pulgar, T., Guzman, M., de Caballos, M.L. Prevention of Alzheimer's disease pathology by cannabinoids: neuroprotection mediated by blockade of microglial activation. J. Neurosci. 2005; 25: 1904–1913.

27. Westlake, T.M., Howlett, A.C., Bonner, T.I., Matsuda, L.A., Herkenham, M. Cannabinoid receptor binding and mRNA expression in human brain: an in vitro autoradiograph and in situ hybridization histochemistry of normal aged and Alzheimer's brains. Neuroscience. 1994; 63: 637–652.

28. Benito, C., Nunez, E., Tolon,R.M., Carrier, E.J., Rabano,A., Hillard, C.J. Cannabinoid CB2 receptors and fatty acid amide hydrolase are selectively overexpressed in neuritic plaque-associated glia in Alzheimer's disease brains. J. Neurosci. 2003; 23: 11136–11141.

29. Wyss-Coray,T. Inflammation in Alzheimer's disease: driving force, bystander or beneficial response. Nat. Med. 2006; 12:1005–1015.

30. Stella,N., Schweitzer, P., Piomelli, D. A second endogenous cannabinoid that modulates long-term potentiation. Nature. 1997; 388: 773–778.

31. Marsicano, G., Goodenough, S., Monory, K., Hermann, H., Eder,M., Cannich,A. et al. CB1 receptors and on-demand defense against excitotoxicity. Science. 2003; 302: 84–88.

32. Van der Stelt, M., Mazzola, C., Espostip, G., Mathias, I., Petrosino,S., DeFilippis, D. et al. Endocannacinoids and Beta-amyloid-induced neurotoxicity in vivo: effect of pharmacological elevation of endocannabinoid levels. Cell. Mol. Life Sci. 2006; 63:1410–1424.

33. Milton,N.G.N. Anandamide and noland ether prevent excitotoxicity of the human amyloid-Beta-peptide, Neurosci. Lett. 2002; 332: 127–130.

34. Castellano, C., Rossi-Arnaud, C., Cestari, V., Costanzi, M. Cannabinoids and memory: animal studies. Curr. Drug Targets CNS Neurol Gisord. 2003; 2: 389–402.

35. Gifford, A.N., Bruneus, M., Gatley, S.J., Volkow, N.D. Cannabinoid receptor-mediated inhibition of acetylcholine release from hippocampal and cortical synaptosomes. Br. J. Pharmacol. 2000; 131: 162–650.

36. Wolff, M.C., Leander, J.D. SR141716A, a cannabinoid CB1 receptor antagonist, improves memory in a delayed radial maze task. Eur. J. Pharmacol. 2003; 477: 213–217.

37. Mazzola, C., Micale, V., Drago, F. Amnesia induced by beta-amyloid fragments in counteracted by cannabinoid CB1 receptor blockabe. Eur. J. Pharmacol. 2003; 477: 219–225.

38. Smith, I.F., Green, K.N., LaFerla, F.M. Calcium disregulation in Alzheimer's disease: recent advances gained from genetically modified animals. Cell. Calcium. 2005; 38: 427–437.

39. Sonkusare, S.K., Kaul, C.L., Ramarao, P. Dementia of Alzheimer's disease and other neurodegenerative disorders-memantine, a new hope. Pharmacol, Res. 2005; 51: 1–17.

40. Rose, C.R., Konnerth, A., Stores not just for storage, intracellular release and synaptic plasticity. Neuron. 2001; 1: 519–522.

41. MacManus, A., Ramsden, M., Murray, M., Pearson, H.A., Campbell,V. Enhancement of 45Ca2+ influx and voltage-dependent Ca2+ channel activity by Beta-amyloid (1–40) in rat cortical synaptosomes and cellular cortical neurons: modulation by the pro-inflammatory cytokine interleukin-1Beta. J. Biol. Chem. 2000; 275: 4713–4718.

42. Arispe, N., Pollard, H.B., Rojas,E. Giant multilevel cation channels formed by Alzheimers disease Beta-amyloid 1–40 in bilayer membranes. Proc. Natl. Acad. Sci. USA 1993; 90: 10573–10577.

43. Nadler, V., Mechoulam, R., Sokolovsky, M. The non-psychotrophic cannabinoid (+)-3S,4S)-7-hydroxy-Delta 6- tetrahydrocannabinol1,1-dimethylheptyl (HU-211) attenuates N-methyl-D-aspartate receptor-mediated neurotoxicity in primary cultures of rat forebrain. Neurosci. Lett. 1993; 162: 43–45.

44. Mackie, K., Hille, B. Cannabinoids inhibit N-type calcium channels in neuroblastoma-glioma cell lines. Proc. Natl. Acad Sci. USA. 1992; 89: 3825–3829.

45. Twitchell, W., Brown, S., Mackie, K. Cannabinoids inhibit N- and P/Q-type calcium channels in cultured rat hippocampal neurons, J. Neurophysiol. 1997; 78: 43–50.

46. Shen, M., Thayer, S.A. Cannabinoid receptor agonist protect cultured mouse hippocampal neurons from excitotoxicity. Brain. Res. 1998; 783: 77–84.

47. Takahashi,K. A., Castillo, P. E. CB1 cannabinoid receptor mediates glutaminergic synaptic suppression in the hippocampus. Neuroscience. 2006; 139: 795–802.

48. Wang, S.J. Cannabinoid CB1 receptor-mediated inhibition of glutamate release from rat hippocampal synaptosomes. Eur. J. Pharmacol. 2003; 469: 47–55.

49. DiMarzo,V., Fontana, A., Cadas,H., Schinell, S., Clmlno, G., Schwartz, J. et al. Formation and inactivation of endogenous cannabinoid anandamide in central neurons. Nature. 1994; 372: 686–691.

50. Hansen, H.H., Ikonomidou, C., Bittigau,P., Hansen, S.H., Hansen, H.S. Accumulation of the anandamide precursor and other N-acetylethanolamine phospholipids in infant rat models of in vivo necrotic and apoptotic neuronal death. J. Neurochem. 2001; 76: 39–46.

51. Zhuang, S-Y., Bridges,D., Grigoenko, E., McCloud, S., Boon, A., Hampson, R.E., et al. Cannabinoids produce neuroprotection by reducing intracellular calcium release from ryanodine-sensitive stores. Neuropharmcology. 2005; 28: 1086–1096.

52. Kim, S. H., Won, S.J., Mao, A., Ledent, C., Jin, K., Greenberg, D.A. Role for neuronal nitric-oxide synthase in cannabinoid-induced neurogenegis. J. Pharmacol. Exp. Ther. 2006; 319: 150–154.

53. Khaspekov, L.G., Brenz, Verca, M.S., Frumkina, L.E., Herman, H., Marsicano, G., Lutz, B. Involvement of brain-derived neurotrophic factor in cannabinoid receptor-dependent protection against excitotoxicity. Eur. J. Neurosci. 2004; 19: 1691–1698.

54. Sanchez, M.G., Ruiz-Llorente, L., Sanchez, A.M., Diaz-Laviada, I. Activation of phosphoinositol 3-kinase/PKB pathway by CB1 and CB2 cannabinoid receptors expressed in prostate PC-3 cells. Involvement in Raf-1 stimulation and NGF induction. Cell. Signal. 2003; 15: 851–859.

55. Hampson, A.J., Grimaldi, M., Axelrod, J., Wink, D. Cannabidiol and (-)Delta9-tetrahydrocannabinol are neuroprotective antioxidants. Proc. Natl. Acad. Sci. USA. 1998; 95: 8268–8273.

56. Esposito, G., DeFilipps, D., Maiuri, M.C., DeStefano, D., Carnuccio, R., Ivuone, T.

Cannabidiol inhibits inducible NOS expression and NO production in Beta-amyloid-stimulated PC12 neurons through p38 MAP kinase and NFkappaB involvement. NEUROSCI. LETT. 2006; 399: 91.

57. Iuvone, T., Esposito,G., Esposito, R., Santamaria, R., DiRosa, M., Izzo, A.A. Neuroprotective effect of cannabidiol, a non-psychoactive component from Cannabis sativa, on Beta-amyloid-induced toxicity in PC12 cells. J. Neurochem. 2004; 89: 134–141.

58. Esposito,G.,DeFilippis,D.,Carnuccio,R.,Izzo, A.G., Iuvone, T. The marijuana component, cannabidiol, inhibits Beta-amyloid-induced tau protein hyperphosphorylation through Wnt/Beta-catenin pathway rescue in PC12 cells. J. Mol. Med. 2006; 84: 253–258.

59. Phiel,C.J., Wilson, C.A., Lee, V.M., Klein, P.S. GSK3 regulates production of Alzheimer's disease Beta-amyloid peptides. Nature. 2003; 423: 435–439.

60. Fernandez-Ruis, J., Romero, J., Velasco, G., Tolon, R.M., Ramos, J.A., Guzman, M. Cannabinoid CB2 receptor: a new target for controlling neural cell survival. Trends Pharm. Sci.. 2007; 28: 39–45.

61. Ehrhart, J., Obergon, D., Mri, T., Hou, H., Sun, N., Bai, Y., et al. Stimulation of CB2 supresses microglial activation. J. Neuroinflamm. 2005; 12: 22–29.

62. Facchinetti, F., DelGiudice, E., Furegato, S., Passarotto, M., Leon, A. Cannabinoids abate release of TNF-alpha in rat microglial cells stimulated with lipopolysaccharide. Glia. 2003; 41: 161–168.

63. Panikashvili, D., Mechoulam, R., Beni, S.M., Alexandrovich, A., Shohami, E. CB1 cannabinoid receptors are involved in neuroprotection via NFxB. Blood Flow Metab. 2005; 25: 477–484.

64. Molina-Holgado, F., Pinteaux, E., Moore, J.D., Molina-Holgado, E., Guaza, C. Gibson, R.M., et al. Endogenous interleukin-1 receptor antagonist mediates anti-inflammatory and neuroprotective actions of cannabinoids in neurons and glia. J. Neurosci. 2003; 12: 6470–6474.

65. Pertwee, R.G. Pharmacological actions of cannabinoids. Handb. Exp. Pharmacol. 2005; 168: 1–51.

66. Grote, H.E., Hannan, A.J. Regulators of adult neurogenesis in the healthy and diseased brain. Clin. Exp. Pharm. Phys. 2007; 34: 533–545.

67. Dong, H., Goico, B., Martin, M., Csernansky, C.A., Bertchume, A. Csernansky, J.G. Modulation of hippocampal cell proliferation, memory and amyloid plaque deposition in APPsw (Tg2576) mutant mice by isolation stress. Neurosci. 2004; 127: 601–609.

68. Jin, K., Peel, A.l., Mao, X.L., Cottrell, B. Henshall, D.C., et al. Increased hippocampal neurogenesis in Alzheimer's disease. Proc. Natl. Acad. Sci. USA. 2004; 101: 343–347.

69. Lee, J., Duan, W., Long, J.M., Ingram, G.K., Mattson, M.P. Dietary restriction increases the number of newly generated neural cells and induced BDNF expression in the dentate gyrus of rats. J. Mol. Neurosci. 2000; 15: 99–108.

70. Galve-Roperh, I., Aguada, T., Palazuelos, J., Guzman, M. The endocannabinoid system and neurogenesis in health and disease Neuroscientist. 2007; 13: 109–114.

71. Palazuelos, J., Aguado, T., Egia,A., Mechoulam, R., Guzman, M. Galve-Roperh, I. Non-psychoactive CB2 cannabinoid agonist stimulate neural progenitor proliferation. FASEB. J. 2006; 20: 2405–2407

72. Jiang, W., Zhang, Y., Xiao, L., Van Cleemput,J., Bai, G. Cannabinoids promote embryonic and adult hippocampal neurogenesis and produce anxiolytic and anti-depressant-like effects. J. Clin. Invest. 2005; 115: 3104–3116.

73. Interosa, N.C., Alvarez, A., Pecez, C.A., Moreno, R.D., Vicent, M., Linker, C., et al. Acetylcholinesterase accelerates assembly of amyloid-Beta-peptides into Alzheimer's fibrils: possible role of the peripheral site of the enzyme. Neuron. 1996; 16: 881–891.

74. Alvarez, A., Alarcon, A., Opazo,C., Campos, E.O., Munoz, F., alderon, F.H., et al. Stable complexes involving acetylcholinesterase and amyloid-Beta-fibrils chance the biochemical properties of the enzyme and increase the neurotoxicity of Alzheimer's fibrils. J. Newurosci. 1998; 18: 407–416.

75. Esposito, G., Scuderi, C., Savani, C., Steardo, L. Jr., De Filippis,D., et al. Cannabidiol in vivo blunts Beta-amyloid induced neuro-inflammation by suppressing IL-1Beta and

iNOS expression. Br. J. Pharmacol. 2007; 151:1272–1279.

76. Castillo,A., Tolon, M.R., Fernandez-Ruis, J., Romero, J., Martinez-Orgado, J. The neuroprotective effect of cannabidiol in an in vitro model of newborn hypoxic-ischemic brain damage in mice is mediated by CB2 and adenosine receptors. Neurobiol. Dis. 2010; 37: 434–440.

77. O'Sullivan, S.E. Cannabinoids go nuclear evidence for activation of peroxisome proliferator-activated receptors. Br. J. Pharmacol. 2007; 152: 576–582.

78. Kersten, S., Peroxisome proliferator activated receptors and lipoprotein metabolism. PPAR Res. 2008.132960 p.

79. Bensinger, S.J., Tontonaz, P., Integration of metabolism and inflammation by lipid-activated nuclear receptors. Nature. 2008; 454: 470–477.

80. Bookout,A.L., Jeong, Y., Downes, M., Yu, R.T., Evans, R.M., et al. Anatomical profiling of nuclear receptor expression reveals a hiearchia transcriptional network. Cell. 2006; 126: 789–799.

81. De la Monte, S.M., Wands, J.R. Molecular indicies of oxidative stress and mitochondrial dysfunction occur early and often progress with severity of Alzheimer's disease. J. Alzheimers Dis. 2006; 9: 167–181.

82. Mrak, R.E., Griffin, W.S. Interleukin-1, neuroinflammation, and Alzheimer's disease. Neurobiol Aging 2001; 22:903–908

83. Zhang, D., Hu, X., O'Callaghan, JP., Hong, J.S. Astrogliosis in CNS Pathologies: Is there a role for microglia? Mol. Neurobiol. 2010; 41: 232–241.

84. Glass, C.K., Saijo, K., Winner, B., Marchetto, M.C., Gage, F,H. Mechanisms underlying inflammation in neurodegeneration. Cell. 2010; 140: 918–934.

85. Magen, I., Avraham, Y., Ackerman, Z., Vorobiev, L., Mechoulam, R., et al. Cannabidiol ameliorates cognitive and motor impairments in mice with bile duct ligation. J. Hepatol. 2009; 51: 528–534.

86. Magen,I., Avraham,Y., Ackerman, Z., Vorobiev, L., Mechoulam, R., et al. Cannabidiol ameliorates cognitive and motor impairments in bile-duct ligated mice via 5-HT1A receptor activation. Br. J. Pharmacol. 2010; 159: 950–957.

87. Avraham, Y., Grigoriadis, N., Poutahidis, T., Vorobiev, L., Magen, I., et al. Cannabidiol improves brain and liver function in a fulminant hepatic failure-induced model of hepatic encelopathy in mice. Br. J. Pharmacol. 2011; 162: 1650–1658.

88. Bianchi, R., Giambanco, I., Donato, R. S100B/Rage-dependent activation of microglia via NF-kappaB and AP-1 Co-regulation of COX-2 expression by S100B, IL-1Beta and TNF-alpha. Neurobiol. Aging. 2010: 31: 665–677.

89. Esposito, G., Scuderi, C., Lu, J., DeFilippis, D., et al. S100B induces tqu protein hyperphosphorylation via Dickopff-1 up-regulation and disrupts the Wnt pathway in human neural stem cells. J. Cell. Mol. Med. 2008; 12: 914–927.

90. Mori, T., Koyama, N., Arendash, G.W., Horikoshi-Sakuraba, Y., Tan, J, et al. Overexpression of human S100B exacerbates cerebral amyloidosis and gliosis in the Tg2576 mouse model of Alzheimer's disease. Glia. 2010; 58: 300–314.

91. Bright, J.J., Kanakasabai, S., Chearwae, W., Chakraborty, S. PPAR Regulation od inflammatory Signaling in CNS Diseases. PPAR Res. 2008. 658520 p.

92. Landreth, G., Jiang, Q., Mandrekar, S., Heneka,M. PPARgamma agonists as therapeutics for the treatment of Alzheimer's disease. Neurotherapeutics. 2008; 5: 481–489.

93. Bodles, A.M., Barger, S.W. Secreted Beta-amyloid precursor protein activates microglia via JNK and p38-MAPK. Neurobiol. Aging. 2005; 26: 9–16.

94. Ho, G.J., Drego, R., Hakimian, E., Masliah,E. Mechanisms of cell signaling and inflammation in Alzheimer's disease. Curr. Drug Targets Inflamm. Allergy. 2004; 4:247–256.

95. Kapadia, R., Yi,J.H., Vemuganti,R. Mechanisms of anti-inflammatory and neuroprotective actions of PPAR-gamma agonists. Front. Biosci. 2008; 13: 1813–1826.

96. O'Banion, M.K. COX-2 and Alzheimer's disease: Potential roles in inflammation and neurodegeneration. Expert Opin. Invest. Drugs 1999; 8: 1521–1536.

97. Feinstein, D.L. Therapeutic potential of peroxisome proliferator-activated receptor agonists for neurologic disease. Diabetes Tech. Ther. 2003; 5: 67–73.

98. Landreth, G.E., Heneka, M.T. Anti-inflammatory actions of peroxisomes proliferator-activated receptor-gamma agonists in Alzheimer's disease. Neurobio. Aging. 2001; 22: 937–944.

99. Lazarov, ., Marr, R.A. Neurogenesis and Alzheimer's disease: at the crossroads. Exp. Neurol. 2010; 223: 267–281.

100. Abrous, D.N., Koehl, M., LeMoal, M. Adult neurogenesis: from precursors to network and physiology. Physiol. Rev. 2005; 85: 523–569.

101. Mayo, W., Lemaire, V., Malaterre, J., Rodriguez, J.J., Cayre, M., et al. Pregnenolone sulfate enhances neurogenesis and PSA-NCAM in young and aged hippocampus. Neurobiol. Aging. 2005; 26: 103–114.

102. Li, B., Yamamori, H., Tatebayashi, Y., Shafit-Zagardo, B., Tanimukai, H., et al. Failure of neuronal maturation in Alzheimer's disease dentate gyrus. J. Neuropathol. Exp. Neurol. 2008; 67: 78–84.

103. Wada, K., Nakajima, A., Katayama, K., Kudo, C., Shibuya, A., et al. Peroxisome proliferator-activated receptor-gamma-mediated regulation of neural stem cell proliferation and differentiation. J. Biol. Chem. 2006; 281: 12673–12681.

104. Migilo, G., Rattazzi,L., Rosa, A.C., Fantozzi, R. PPAR-gamma stimulation promotes neuritic outgrowth in SH-SY5Y human neuroblastoma cells. Neurosci. Lett. 2009; 454: 134–138.

105. Wolf, S.A., Bick-Sander, A., Fabel, K., Leal-Galicia, P., Tauber, S., et al. Cannabinoid receptor CB1 mediates baseline and activity-induced survival of new neurons in adult hippocampal neurogenesis. Cell. Commun. Signal 2010; 8: 12

106. Duyckaerts, C., Dickson, D. "Neuropathology od Alzheimer's disease and irts variants," in Neurodegeneration: The Molecular Pathology of Dementia ND MOVEMENT DISORDERS, 2ND EDN, Eds D Dickson and R. Weller(West Sussex,Wiley_Blackwell)2011: 62–91.

107. Ferrer, I. Defining Alzheimer as a common age-related neurodegenerative process nor inevitably leading to dementia. Prog. Neurobiol. 2012; 97: 38–51. Doi:10.1016/j.pneurobio.2012.03.005.

108. Bertram, L., Tanzi, R.E. "Genetics of Alzheimer's disease," in Neurodegeneration: The Molecular Pathology of Dementia and Movement Disorders, 2nd Edn, eds D.Dickson and R Weller (West Sussex: Wiley-Blackwell) 2011: 51–91. Doi: 10.1002/9781444341256.ch9

109. Frost, B., Diamond, M.I. Prion-like mechanisms in neurodegenerative diseases. Nat. Rev. Neurosci. 2010; 11: 155–159. Doi:10.1038/nrn2786.

110. Pamplona, R., Dalfo,E., Ayala, V., Bellmunt, M.J., Prat, J. Ferrer, I. et al. Proteins in human brain cortex are modified by oxidation, glycoxidation, and lipoxidation: effects of Alzheimer disease asnd identification of lipoxidation targets. J. Biol. Chem. 2005; 280: 21522–21530. Doi: 10.1074/jbc.M502255200.

111. Ferrer, I. Altered mitochondria, energy metabolism, voltage-dependent anion channel, and lipid rafts converge to exhaust neurons in Alzheimer's disease. J. Bioenerg. Biomembr. 2009; 41: 425–431. Doi: 10.1007/s10863–009-9243–5.

112. Sultana, R., Butterfield, D.A., Role of oxidative stress in the progression of Alzheimer's disease. J. Alzheimers Dis 2010; 19: 341–353. Doi: 10.3233/JAD-2010–1222.

113. Maccarrone, M., Dainese, E., Oddi, S. Intracellular trafficking of anandamide: new concepts for signaling. Trends. Biochem. Sci. 2010; 35: 601–608. Doi: 10.1016/j.tibs.2010.05.008.

114. Tolon, R.M., Nunez, E., Pazos, M.R., Benito, C.m Castill0, A.L., Martinez-Orgado, .A. et al. The activation of cannabinoid CB2 receptors in situ and in vitro Beta-amyloid removal by human macrophages. Brain. Res. 2009; 1283: 148–154. Doi: 10.1016/j.brainres.2009.95.098.

115. Martin-Moreno, A.M., Reigada, D., Ramirez, B.G., Mechoulam, R., et al. Cannabidiol and Other Cannabinoids reduce microglial activation in vitro and in vivo: Relevance to Alzheimer's disease. Mol. Pharmacol. 2011; 79: 964–973.

116. Bisogno, T., DiMarzo, V. The role of the Endocannabinoid System in Alzheimer's Disease: Facts and Hypotheses. Curr. Pharmaceut. Des. 2008; 14:2299–2305.

PARKINSON'S DISEASE

1. Fernandez-Ruis, J.J., Gonzalez, S., Romero, J., Ramos, J.A.Cannabinpoids in neurodegeneration and neuroprotection. Cannabinoids as Therapeutics. 2005. Birkhauser Verlag: Switzerland; 79–109. In; Mechoulam, R. (ed.)

2. Fernandez-Ruis, J., deMiguel, R., Hernandez, M., Cebeira, M., Ramos, J.A. Endocannabinoids and Dopamine-Related Functions in the CNS. Endocannabinoids The Brain and Body's Marijuana and Beyond. 2006 CRC Press, Boca Raton, Fla. 261–290. In: Onaivi, E., Sugiura, T., DiMarzo, V. (ed.)

3. Blandini, F., Nappi, G., Tassoverlli, C., Martignoni, E. Functional changes in the basal ganglia circuitry in Parkinson's disease. Prog. Neurobiol. 2000; 62: 63–88.

4. McGeer, P.L., Yasojima, K., McGeer, E.G. Inflammation in Parkinson's disease. Adv. Neurol. 2001; 86: 83–89.

5. Sherer, T.B., Berarbet, R., Greenamyre,, J.T. Pathogenesis of Parkinson's disease. Curr. Opin. Investig. Drugs. 2001; 2: 657–662.

6. Sethi, K.D. Clinical aspects of Parkinson's disease. Curr. Opin. Neurol. 2002; 15:456–460.

7. Carlsson, A. Treatment of Parkinson's with L-DOPA. The early discovery phase, and a comment on current problems. J. Neurol. Transm. 2002; 109: 777–787.

8. Vajda, F.J. Neuroprotection and neurodegenerative disease. J. Clin. Neurosci. 2002; 9: 4–8.

9. Tintner, R., Jankovic, J. Treatment options for Parkinson's disease. Curr. Opin. Neurol. 2002; 15: 467–476.

10. Fernandez-Ruis, J.J., Lastres-Becker,I., Cabranes, A., Gonzalez, S., Ramos, J.A. Endocannabinoids and basal ganglia functionality. Prost. Leukot. Essent. Fatty Acids. 2002; 66: 263–273.

11. Consroe, P. Brain cannabinoid system as targets for the therapy of neurological disorders. Neurobiol. Dis. 1998; 5: 534–551.

12. Muller-Vahl, K.R., Kolbe, H., Schneider, U., Emrich, H.M. Cannabis in movement disorders. Frosch Komplementarmed. 1999; 6: 23–27.

13. Lastres-Becker, I., Ceberia, M., Ceballos, M., Zeng, B-Y., Jenner, P., Ramos, J.A., Fernandez-Ruis, J.J. Increased cannabinoid CB1 receptor binding and activation of GTP=binding protein in the basal ganglia of patients with Parkinson's disease and MPTP-treated marmosets. Eur. J. Neurosci. 2001; 14:1827–1832.

14. Romero, J., Berrendero,F., Perez-Rosado, A., Manzannres, J, Rojo, A., Fernandez-Ruis.J.J., Yebenes, J.G., Ramos, J.A. Unilateral 6-hydroxydopamine lesions of nigrostriatal dopaminergic neurons increased CB1 receptor mRNA levels I the caudate-putamen. Life. Sci. 2000; 66: 485–494.

15. Maileux, P., Vanderhaeghen, J.J. Dopaminergic regulation of cannabinoid receptor mRNA levels in the rat caudate-putmen: an in situ hybridization study. J. Neurochem. 1993; 61: 1705–1712.

16. Garcia-Arencibia, M., Gonzalez, S., deLago, E., Ramos,J.A., Mechoulam, R., Fernandez-Ruis,J. Evaluation of the neuroprotective effect of cannabinoids in a rat model of Parkinson's disease: importance of antioxidant and cannabinoid receptor-independent properties. Brain Res. 2007; 1134(1): 162–70.

17. Sagredo, O., Ramos, J.A., Decio, A., Mechoulam, R., Fernandez-Ruis, J. Cannabidiol reduced the4 striatal atrophy caused by 3-notropropionic acid in vivo by mechanisms independent of the activation of cannabinoid, Vanilloid TRPV1 and adenosine receptors. Eur. J. Neurosci. 2007; 26(4): 843–51.

18. Herman,D., Sartorius, A., Welzel, H., Walter, S., Skopp, G., Ende, G., Mann, K. Dorsolateral prerontal cortex N-acteylaspartate/total

creatine (NAA/tCr) loss in male recreational cannabis users. Biol. Psychiatry. 2007; 61(11):1281–9.

19. Zuardi, A.W., Crippa, J.A.S., Hallak, J.E.C., Pinto, J.P., Nisihara, M.H.C., Rodrigues, G.G.R., Dursum, S.M., Tumas, V. Cannabidiol fot the treatment of psychosis in Parkinson's disease: possible mechanisms of actions. J. Psychopharmacol. 2009; 23(8): 979–83.

20. Iuvone,T., Esposito,G., Esposito, R., Santamaria, R., DiRosa, M., Izzo, A.A. Neuroprotective effect of cannabidiol, a non-psychoactive component from Cannabis sativa, on Beta-amyloid-inducwed toxicity in PC12 cells. J. Neurochem. 2004; 89(1): 134–41.

21. Zhang,P., Tian, B. Metabolic Syndrome: An im[portant risk factor for Parkinson's disease. Oxid. Med. And Cell. Long. Vol2014(2014), Article ID 729194. Doi:10.1155/2014/729194 http://www.hindawi.com/journals/omcl/2014/729194/

22. Abbott, A.H., Serdula, M.K., Dietz, W.H., Bowman, B.A., Marks, J.S., Koplan, J.P. "Midlife adiposity and the future risk of Parkinson's disease." Neurology. 2002; 59(7): 1051–57.

23. Whitmer, R.A., Gunderson, E.P., Barrett-Connor, E., Quesenberry, Jr., C.P., Yaffe, K. "Obesity in middle age and future risk of dementia: a 27 year longitudinal population based study." Br Med. J. 2005; 330(7504):1360–62.

24. Hu, G., Jousilahti, P., Nissinen, A., Antikainen, R., Kivipelto, M., Tuomilehto, J. "Body mass index and the risk of Parkinson's disease." Neurology. 2006; 67(11): 1955–59.

25. Morris, J.K., Bomhoff, G.L., Stanford, J.A., Geiger, P.C. "Neurodegeneration in an animal model of Parkinson's disease id exacerbated by a high fat diet." Amer. J. Physiol-Reg. Integrative and Comp. Physiol. 2010; 299(4): R1082-R1090.

26. Choi, J.Y., Jang, E.H., Park, C.S., Kang, J.H. "Enhanced susceptibility to 1-methyl-4-phenyl-1,2,3,6-tetrahydropyridine neurotoxicity in high-fat diet-induced obesity." Free Radical Biol. and Med. 2005; 38(6): 806–16.

27. Cano, P., Cardinali, D.P., Rios-Lugo, M.J., Fernandez-Mateos, M.P., Reyes Toso, C.F., Esquifino, A.I. "Effect of a high-fat diet on 24-hour pattern of circulating adipocytokines in rats." Obesity. 2009; 17(10): 1866–1871.

28. Gupye,A.A., Bomhoff, G.L., Swerdlow, R.H., Geiger, P.C. "Heat treatment improves glucose tolerance and prevents skeletal muscle insulin resistance in rats fed a high-fat diet." Diabetes. 2009; 58(3): 567–578.

29. Uranga, R.M., Bruce-Keller, A.J., Morrison, C.D. et al. "Intersection between metabolic dysfunction, high fat diet consumption, and brain aging." J. Neurochem. 2010; 114(2): 344–61.

30. Tsuruta, R., Fujita, M., Ono,T. et al. "Hyperglycemia enhances excessive superoxide anion radical generation, oxidative stress, early inflammation, and endothelial injury in forebrain ischmia/reperfusion rats." Brain Res. 2010; 1309: 155–63.

31. Obrosova, I.G., Drel, V.R., Pacher, P. et al. "Oxidative-nitrosative stress and poly(ADP-ribose) polymerase (PARP) activation in experimental diabetic neuropathy: the relation idd revisited." Diabetes. 2005; 54(12): 3435–3441.

32. Szabo,C. "Multiple pathways of peroxynitrite cytotoxicity." Toxicol. Lett. 2003; 140–141: 105–112.

33. Vincent, A.M., Edwards, J.L., Sadadi, M., Feldman, E.L. The antioxidant response as a drug target in diabetic neuropathy. Curr. Drug Targets. 2008; 9(1): 94–109.

34. Allen, D.A., Yaqoob, M.M., Harwood, S.M. Mechanisms of high-glucose induced apoptosis and its relationship to diabetic complications. J. Nutrit. Biochem.. 2005; 16(12): 705–13.

35. Tomlinson, D.R., Gardiner, N.J. Glucose neurotoxicity. Nature Reviews Neurosci. 2008; 9(1): 36–45.

36. Hu, G., Jousilahti, P., Bidel, S., Antikainen, R., Tumilehto, J. Type 2 diabetes and the risk of Parkinson's disease. Diabetes Care. 2007; 30(4): 842–47.

37. Woo, K.S., Chook, P., Lolin, Y.I. et al. Hyperhomocyst(e)inemia is a risk factor for arterial endothelial dysfunction in humans. Circulation. 1997; 96: 2542–44.

38. Kruman, I.I., Culmsee, C., Chan, S.L. et al. Homocysteine elicits a DNA damage response

in neurons that promotes apoptosis and hypersensitivity to excitotoxicity. J. Neurosci. 2000; 20918): 6920–26.

39. Gomes Trolin, C., Regland, B., Oreland, L. Decreased methionine adenosyltransferase activity in erythrocytes of patients with dementia disorders. Eur. Neuropsychopharmacol. 1995; 5(2): 107–14.

40. Blandini, F., Fancellu, R., Martignoni, E. et al. Plasma homocysteine and L-DOPA metabolism in patients with Parkinson's disease. Clin. Chem. 2001; 47(6): 1102–04.

41. Bottiglieri, T., Hyland, K. S-adenosylmethionine levels in psychiatric and neurological disorders: a review. Acta Neurologica Scandinavica, Supplement. 1994; 89(154): 19–26.

42. Loscalzo, J. Yhe oxidant stress of hyperhomocyst(e)inemia. The J. Clin. Investig. 1996; 98(1): 5–7.

43. Kurz, K., Frick, B., Furhapter,C. et al. Homocysteine metabolism in different human cells. Issues. 2013, 24.

44. McGeer, P.L., Itagaki, S., Boyes, B.E., McGeer, E.G. Reactive microglia are positive for HLA-dr in the substancia nigra of Parkinson's and Alzheimer's disease patients. Neurology. 1988; 38(8): 1285–91.

45. Whitton, P.S. Inflamation as a causative factor in the aetiology of Parkinson's disease. Br. J. Pharmacol. 2007; 150(8): 963–76.

46. Tansey, M.G., Frank-Cannon, T.C., McCoy, M. K. et al. Neuroinflammation in Parkinson's disease: is there sufficient evidence for mechanism-based interventional therapy. Front. Biosci. 2008; 13(2): 709–17.

47. Mogi, M., Harada, M., Kondob, T. et al. Interleukin-1Beta, interleukin-6, epidermal growth factor and transforming growth factor-alpha are elevated in the brain from parkinsonian patients. Neurosci. Lett. 1994; 180(2): 147–50.

48. Blum-Degena, D., Muller, T., Kuhn, W., erlach, M., Przuntek, H., Riedserer, P. Intwerleukin-1beta and interleukin-6 are elevated in the cerebrospinal fluid of Alzheimer's and de novo Parkinson's patients. Neurosci. Lett. 1995; 202(1–2): 17–20.

49. Muller, T., Blum-Degen, D., Przuntek, H., Kuhn, W. Interleukin-6 levels in cerebrospinal fluid inversely correlate to severity of Parkinson's disease. Acta Neuroogica Scandinavica. 1998; 98(2): 142–44.

50. Imai, Y., Soda, M., Inoue, H., Hattori, N., Mizuno, Y., Takahashi, R. An unfolded putative transmembrane polypeptide, which can lead to endoplasmic reticulum stress, is a substrate of Parkin. Cell. 2001; 105(7): 891–902.

51. Imai,Y., Soda, M., Hatakeyama, s. et al. CHIP is associated with Parkin, a gene responsible for famlil Parkinson's disease, and enhances its ubiquitin ligase activity. Molecular Cell 2002; 10(1): 55–67.

52. Kaufman, R.J. Orchestrating the unfolded protein response in health and disease. J. Clin. Investig. 2002; 110(10): 1389–98.

53. Imai,Y., Soda, M., Takahashi,R. Parkin suppresses unfolded protein stress-induced cell death theough its E3 ubiquitin-protein ligase activity. J. Biol. Chem. 2000; 275(46): 35661–664.

54. Bournival, J., Quessy, P., Martinoli, M. Protective effects of resveratrol and quercetin against MPP+ induced oxidative stress act by modulating markers of apoptotic death in dopaminergic neurons. Cell. Molec. Neurobiol. 2009; 29(8): 1169–80.

55. Bournival, J., Francoeur, M.A., Renaud, J., Martinoli, M.G. Quercetin and sesamin protect neuronal PC12 cells from high-glucose-induuced oxidation, nitrosive stress, and apoptosis. Rejuvenation Research. 2012; 15(3): 322–33.

56. Bureau, G., Longpre, zf., Martinoli, M. Resveratrol and quercetin, two natural polyphenols, reduce apoptotic neuronal cell death induced by neuroinflammation. J. Neurosci. Res. 2008; 86(2): 403–10.

57. Aruoma, O.I., Hayashi, Y., Marotta, F., Mantello, P., Rachmilewitz, E., Montagnier, L. Applications and bioefficacy of the functional food supplement fermented papaya preparation. Toxicology. 2010; 278(1): 6–16.

58. Cao,H., Oin, B., Panickar, K.S., Anderson, R.A. Tea and cinnamon polyphenols improve the metabolic syndrome. Argo Food Industry Hi-Tech. 2008; 19(6): 14–17.

59. Gelinas, S., Martinoli, M. Neuroprotective effect of estradiol and phytoestrogens on MPP+-induced cytotoxicity in neuronal PC12 cells. J. Neurosci. Res. 2002; 70(1): 90–96.

60. Garcia-Arencibia, M., Gonzales, S., deLago, E., Ramos, J.A., Mechoulam, R. Fernandez-Ruiz, J. Evaluation of the neuroprotective effect of cannabinoids in a rat model of Parkinson's disease: importance of antioxidant and cannabinoid receptor-independent properties. Brain Res. 2007; 1134(1): 162–70.

61. Booz, G.W. Cannabidiol as an emergent therapeutic strategy for lessening the impact of inflammation on oxidative stress. Free Radical Biol. and Med. 2011; 51(5): 1054–61.

62. Pacher, P., Batkai, S., Kunos, G. The endocannabinoid system as an emerging target of pharmacotherapy. Pharmacol. Rev. 2006; 58(3): 389–462.

63. Winquist,A., Streenland,K., Shankar,A. Higher serum uric acid associated with decreased Parkinson's disease prevalence in a large Community-based survey. Movement Disorders. 2010; 25(7): 932–36.

64. Andreadou,E., Nikolaou,C., Gournaras, F. et al. Serum uric acid levels in patients with Parkinson's disease: their relationship to treatment and disease duration. Clin Neurol. And Neurosurg. 2009; 111(9): 724–28.

65. Alvarez-Lario, B., Macaroon-vincent,J. Is there anything good in uric acid? QJM 2011; 104(12): 1015–24, Article ID hcr159

66. Chen, H., Mosley, T.H., Alonso,A.., Huang, X. Plasma urate and Parkinson's disease in the atherosclerosis risk in communities (ARIC) study. Am. J. Epidemiology. 2009; 169(9): 1064–69.

67. Huang, C.S., Kawamura, T., Toyoda, Nakao, A. Recent advances in hydrogen research as a therapeutic medical gas. Free Radical Research. 2010; 44(9): 971–82.

68. Fujita,K., Seike, T., Yutsudo, N. et al. Hydrogen in drinking water reduces dopaminergic neuronal loss in the 1-methyl-4-phenyl-1,2,3,6-Tetrahydropyridine mouse model of Parkinson's disease. PLoS ONE. 2009; 4(9), Article ID e7247

69. Fu, Y., Ito,M., Fujita,Y. et al. Molecular hydrogen is protective against 6-hydroxydopamine-induced nigrostriatal degeneration in a rat model of Parkinson's disease. Neurosci. Lett. 2009; 453(2): 81–85.

70. Ohsawa, I., Ishikawa,M., Takahashi, K. et al. Hydrogen acts as a therapeutic antioxidant by selectively reducing cytotoxic oxygen radicals. Nature Medicine. 2007; 13(6): 688–94.

71. Ross, G.W., Abbott, R.D., Petrovitch, H. et al. Association of coffee and caffeine intake with the risk of Parkinson's disease. JAMA. 2000; 283(20): 2674–79.

72. Nehlig, A., Daval, J. L., Debry, G. Caffeine and the central nervous system: mechanisms of action, biochemical, metabolic and psychostimulant effects. Brain Research Rev. 1992; 17(2): 139–69.

73. Popoli,P., Caporali, M.G., Scotti de Carolis, A. Akinesia due to catecholamine depletion in mice is prevented by caffeine. Further evidence for an involvement of adenosinergic system in the control of motility. J. Pharmacy and Pharmacol. 1991; 43(4): 280–81.

74. Daly, J.W. Caffeine analogs: biomedical impact. Cellular and Molecular Life Sciences. 2007; 64(16): 2153–69.

75. Decasagayam, T.P., Kamat, J. P., Mohan, H., Kesavan, P.C. Caffeine as an antioxidant: inhibition of lipid peroxidation induced by reactive oxygen species. Biochimica et Biophysica Acta. 1996; 1282: 63–70.

76. Knekt, P., Kilkkinen, A., Rissanen, H., Marniemi, J., Saaksjarvi, K., Heliovaara, M. Serum vitamin D aand the risk of Parkinson's disease. Archives of Neurology. 2010; 67(7): 808–11.

77. Buell, J.S., Dawson-Hughes, B. Vitamin D and neurocognitive dysfunction: preventing "D"ecline? Molecular Aspects of Medicine. 2008; 29(6): 415–22.

78. Newmark, H.L., Newmark, J. Vitamin D and Parkinson's disease-a hypothesis. Movement Disorders. 2007; 22(4): 461–68.

79. Eyles, D.W., Smith,S., Kinobe, R., Hewison, M., McGrath, J.J. Distribution of the Vitamin D receptor and 1 alpha-hydroxylase in human brain. J. Chem. Neuroanatomy. 2005; 29(1): 21–30.

80. Liou, G.I., Auchampach, J.A., Hillard, C.J., Zhu, G., Yousufzai, B., Mian, S., Khan, S., Khalifa, Y. Medication od cannabidiol anti-

inflammation in the retina by equilibrative nucleoside transporter and A2A adenosine receptor. Investig. Ophthalmol. Vis. Sci. 2008; 49: 5526–5531.

81. Carrier, E.J., Auchampach, J.A., Hillard, C.J. Inhibition of an equilibrative nucleoside transporter by cannabidiol: a mechanism of cannabinoid immuniosupression. Proc. Natl. Acad. Sci. USA. 2006; 103: 7895–7900.

82. Booz, G.W. Cannabidiol as an emergent therapeutic strategy for lessening the impact of inflammation on oxidative stress. Free Radical Biol. & Med. 2011; 51: 1054–61.

83. Rajesh, M., Mukhopadhyay, P., Batkai, S., Hasko, G. et al. Cannabidiol attenuates high glucose-induced endothelial cell inflammatory response and barrier disruption. Am. J. Physiol. Heart Circ. Physiol. 2007; 293: H610-H619.

84. Moore, D.J., West, A.B., Dawson, V.L., Dawson, T.M. Molecular pathophysiology of Parkinson's disease. Annu. Rev. Neurosci. 2005; 28: 57–87.

85. Izzo, A.A., Borrelli, F., Capasso, R., DiMarzo, V., Mechoulam, R. Non-psychotropic plant cannabinoids: new therapeutic opportunities from an ancient herb. Trends Pharmacol. Sci. 2009; 30: 515–527.

86. Uversky, V.N. A protein-chameleon: conformational plasticity of alpha-synuclein, a disordered protein involved in neurodegenerative disrders. J. Biomol. Struct. Dyn. 2003; 21: 211–34.

87. Irizarry, M.C., Kim, T.W., McNamara, M., Tanzi, R.E., George, J.M. et al. Characterization of the precursor protein of the non-A beta component of senile plaques (NACP) in the human central nervous system. J. Neuropath. Exp. Neurol. 1996; 55: 889–95.

88. Fortin, D.L., Troyer, M.D., Nakamura, K., Kubo, S., Anthony, M.D., Edwards, R.H. Lipid rafts mediate the synaptic localization of alpha-synuclein. J. Neurosci. 2004; 24: 6715–23.

89. Abeliovich, A., Schmitz, Y., Farinas, I., Choi-Lundberg, D., Ho, W.H. Mice lacking alpha-synuclein display functional deficits in the nigrostriatal dopamine system. Neuron. 2000; 25: 239–52.

90. Davidson, W.S., Jonas, A., Clayton, D.F., George, J.M. Stabilization of alpha-synuclein secondairy structure upon binding to synthetic membranes, J. Biol. Chem. 1998; 273: 9443–49.

91. Jenco, J.M., Rawlingson, A., Daniels, B., Morris, A.J. Regulation of phospholipase D2: selective inhibition of mammalian phospholipase D isoenzymes by Alpha- and Beta-synucleins. Biochem. 1998; 37: 4901–9.

92. Cole, N.B., Murphy, D.D., Grider, T., Brasemle, D., Nussbaum, R.L., Lipid droplet binding and oligomerization properties of the Parkinson's disease protein alpha-synuclein. J. Biol. Chem. 2002; 277: 6344–52.

93. Murphy, D.D., Rueter, S.M., Trojanowski, J.Q., Lee, V.M. Synucleins are developmentally expressed, and alpha-synuclein regulates the size of the presynaptic vesicular pool in primary hippocampal neurons, J. Neurosci. 2000; 20: 3214–20.

94. Conway, K.A., Harper, J.D., Lansbury, P.T. Accelerated in vitro fibril formation by a mutant alpha-synuclein linked to early-onset Parkinson's disease. Nat. Med. 1998; 4: 1318–20.

95. Conway, K.A., Lee, S.J., Rochet, J.C., Ding, T.T., Williamson, R.E., Lansbury, P.T. Jr. Acceleration of oligomerization, not fibrilliation, is a shared property of both alpha-synuclein mutations linked to early-onset Parkinson's disease: implications for pathogenesis and therapy. Proc. Natl. Acad, Sci. USA. 2000; 97: 571–76.

96. Lashuel, H.A., Hartley, D., Petre, B.M., Lansbury, P.T. Jr. Neurodegenerative disease: amyloid pores from pathogenic mutations Nature. 2002; 418:291.

97. Conway, K.A., Rochet, J.C., Bieganski, R.M., Lansbury, P.T. Jr. Kinetic stabilization of the alpha-synuclein protofibril by a dopamine-alpha-synuclein adduct. Science. 2001; 294: 1346–49.

98. Masliah, E., Rockenstein, E., Veinbergs, I., Mallory, M., Hashimoto, M. et al. Dopaminergic loss and inclusion body formation in alpha-synuclein mice: implications for neurodegenerative disorders. Science. 2000; 287: 1265–69.

99. Feaney, M.B., Bender, W.W. A Drosophila model of Parkinson's disease. Nature. 2000; 404: 394–98.

100. Kahle, P.J., Neuman, M. Ozmen, L., Muller, V., Odoy, S. et al. Selective insolubility of alpha-synuclein in human Lewy body diseases is recapitulated in a transgenic mouse model. Am. J. Pathol. 2001; 159: 2215–25.

101. Neumann, M., Kahle, P.J., Giasson, B.I., Ozmen, L., Borroni, E. et al. Misfolded proteinase K-resistant hyperphosphorylated alpha-synuclein in aged transgenic mice with locomotor deterioration and in human alpha-synucleinopathies. J. Clin. Invest. 2002; 110: 1429–39.

102. Betarbet, R., Sherer, T.B., MacKenzie, G., Garcia-Osuna, M., Panov, A.V., Greenamyre, J.T. Chronic systemic pesticide exposure reproduces features of Parkinson's disease. Nat. Neurosci. 2000; 3: 1301–6.

103. Manning-Bog, A.B., McCormack, A.L., Li, J., Uversky, V.N., Fink, A.L., DiMonte, D.A. The herbicide paraquat causes up-regulation and aggregation of alpha-synuclein in mice: parquat and alpha-synuclein. J. Biol. Chem. 2002; 277: 1641–44.

104. Sherewr, T.B., Betarbet, R., Stout, A.K., Lund, S., Baptisa, M. et al. An in vitro model of Parkinson's disease: linking mitochondrial impairment to altered alpha-synuclein metabolism and oxidative damage. J. Neurosci. 2002; 22: 706–15.

105. Sherer, T.B., Kim, J.H., Betarbet, R., Greenamyre, J.T. Subcutaneous rotenone exposure causes highly selective dopaminergic degeneration and alpha-synuclein aggregation. Exp. Neurol. 2003; 179: 9–16.

106. Ischiropoulos, H., Beckman, J.S. Oxidative stress and nitritation in neurodegeneration: cause, effect, or association? J. Clin. Invest. 2003; 111:163–69.

107. Giassson, B.I., Duda, J.E., Murray, A.V., Chen, Q., Souza, J.M. et al. Oxidative damage linked to neurodegeneration by selective alpha-synuclein nitration in synucleinopathy lesions. Science. 2000; 290:985–89.

108. Hodara, R., Norris, .., iasson, B.I., Mishizen-Eberz, A.J., Lynch, D.R. et al. Functional consequences of alpha-synuclein tyrosine nitration: diminished binding to lipid vesicles and increased fibrillar formation J. Biol. Chem. 2004; 279: 47746–53.

109. Li, W., Lesuisse, C., Xu, Y., Tronosco, J.C., Price, D.L., Lee, M.K. Stabilization of alpha-synuclein protein with aging and familial Parkinson's disease-linked A53T mutation. J. Neurosci. 2004; 24: 9400–9.

110. McNaught, K.S., Perl, D.P., Brownell, A.L., Olanow, C.W. Systemic exposure to proteasome inhibitors cause a progressive model of Parkinson's disease. Ann. Neurol. 2004; 56: 149–62.

111. Masliah, E., Rockenstein, E., Veinsburg <i., Sagara, Y., Malloy, M. et al Beta-amyoid peptides enhance alpha-snuclein accumulation and neuronal defects in a transgenic mouse model linking Alzheimer's disease and Parkinson's disease. Proc. Natl, Acad, Sci. USA. 2001; 98: 12245–50.

112. Giasson, B.I., Forman, M.S., Higuchi, M., Golbe, L.I., raves, C.L., et al. Initiation and synergistic fibrillization of tau and alpha-synuclein. Science. 2003; 300: 636–40.

113. Bennett, M.C., Bishop, J.F., Leng, Y., Chock, P.B., Chase, T.N., Mouradian, M.M. Degredation of alpha-synuclein by proteasome. J. Biol. Chem. 1999; 274: 33855–58.

114. Lindersson, E, Beedholm, R., Horjrup, P., Moos, T., Gai, W., et al. Proteasomal inhibition by alpha-synuclein filaments and oligomers. J. Biol. Chem. 2004; 279: 12924–34.

115. Snyder, H., Mwnsah, K., Theisler, C., Lee, J., Matouschek, A., Wolozin, B. Aggregated and momomeric alpha-synuclein bind to the S6' proteasomal protein and inhibit proteasomal function. J. Biol. Chem. 2003; 278: 11753–59.

116. Hsu, L.J., Sagara, Y., Arroyo, A., Rockenstein, E., Sisk, A., et al. Alpha-synuclein promotes mitochondrial deficit and oxidative stress. Am. J. Pathol. 2000; 157: 401–10.

117. Gosavi, N., Lee, H.J., Lee, J.S., Patel, S., Lee, S.j. Golgi fragmentation occurs in

the cells with prefibrillar alpha-synuclein aggregates and preceeds the formation of fibrillar inclusi0ns. J. Biol. Chem. 2002; 277: 48984–92.

118. Lee, M., Hyun, D., Halliwell, B., Jenner, P. Effect of the overexpression of wild-type or mutant alpha-synuclein on cell susceptibility to insult. J. Neurochem. 2001; 76: 998–1009.

119. Cuervo, A.M., Stefanis, L., Fredenburg, R., Lansbury, P.T., Sulzer, D. Impaired degradation of mutant alpha-synuclein by chaperone-mediated autophagy. Science 2004; 305: 1292–95.

120. Ko, L., Mehta, N.D., Farrer, M., Easson, C., Hussey, J., et al. Sensitization of neuronal cells to oxidative stress with mutated human alpha-synuclein. J. Neurochem. 2000; 75: 2546–54.

121. Tabrizi, S.J., Orth, M., Wilkinson, J.M., Taanman. J.W., Warnwer, T.T., et al. Expression of mutant alpha-synuclein causes increased susceptibility to dopamine toxicity. Hum. Mol. Genet. 2000; 9: 2683–89.

122. Lee, F.J., Liu, F., Pristupa, Z.B., Niznik, H.B. Direct binding and functional coupling of alpha-synuclein to the dopamine transporters accelerate dopamine-induced apoptosis. FASEB. J. 2001; 15:916–26.

123. Lotharis, J., Barg, S., Wiekop, P., Lundberg, C., Raymon, H.K., Brundin, P. Effect of mutant alpha-synuclein on dopamine homeostasis in a new human mesencephalic cell line. J. Biol. Chem. 2002; 277: 38884–94.

124. Matsumine, H., Saito, M., Shimonda-Matsubayashi, S., Tanaka, H., Ishikawa, A., et al. Localization of a gene for an autosomal recessive form of juvenile Parkinsonism to chromosome 6q25.2–27. Am. J. Hum. Genet. 1997; 60: 588–96.

125. Kitada, T., Asakawa, S., Hattori, N., Matsumine, H., Yamamura, Y., et al. Mutations in the parkin gene cause autosomal recessive juvenile parkinsonism. Nature. 1998; 392: 605–8.

126. Lucking, C.B., Durr, A., Bonifati, V., Vaughan, J., DeMichele, G., et al. Association between early-onset Psrkinson's

disease and mutations in the parkin gene. French Parkinson's Disease Genetics Study Group. New Engl. J. Med. 2000; 342: 1560–67.

127. Scott, W.K., Nance, M.A., Watts, R.L., Hubble, J.P., Koller, W.C., et al. Complete genomic screen in Parkinson's disease: evidence for multiple genes. JAMA. 2001; 286: 2239–44.

128. Shimura, H. Hattori, N., Kubo, S., Mizuno, Y., Asakawa, S., et al. Famillial Parkinson's disease gene product, parkin, is a ubiquitin-protein ligase. Nat. Genet. 2000; 25: 302–5.

129. Zhang, Y., Gao, J., Chung, K.K., Huang, H., Dawson, V.L., Dawson, Y.M. Parkin function as an E2-dependent ubiquitin-protein ligase and promotes the degredation of the synaptic vesicle-associated protein, CDCrel-1. Proc. Natl. Acad. Sci. USA. 2000; 97: 13354–59.

130. Glickman, M.H., Ciechanover, A. The ubiquitin-proteasome proteolytic pathway: destruction for the sake of construction. Physiol. Rev. 2002; 82: 373–428.

131. Chung, K.K., Zhang, Y., Lim, K.L., Tanaka, Y., Huang, H., et al. Parkin ubiquinates the alpha-synuclein-interacting protein, synphilin-1; implications for Lewybody formations in Parkinson's disease. Natl. ed. 2001; 7: 1144–50.

132. Shimura, H., Schlossmacher, M.G., Hattori, N., Frosch, M.P., Trockenbacher, A., et al. Ubiquination of a new form of alpha-synuclein by parkin from human brain: implications for Parkinson's disease. Science. 2001; 293: 263–69.

133. Imai, Y., Soda, M., Inoue, H., Hattori, N., Mizuno, Y., Takahashi, R. An unfolded putative transmembrane polypeptide, which can lead to endoplasmic reticulum stress, is a substrate of Parkin. Cell. 2001; 105: 891–902.

134. Huynh, D.P., Scoles, D.R., Nguyen, D., Pulst, S.M. The autosomal recessive juvenile Parkinson disease gene product, parkin, interacts with and ubiquinates synaptotagmin XI. Hum. Mol. Genet. 2003; 12: 2587–97.

135. Staropoli, J.F., McDermott, C., Martinat, C., Schulman, B., Demireva, E.,

Abeliovich, A. Parkin is a component of an SCF-like ubiquitin ligase complex and protects postmitotic neurons from kainite excitotoxicity. Neuron. 2003; 37: 735–49.

136. Corti, O., Hampe, C., Koutnikova, H., Darios, F., Jacquer, S., et al. The p38 subunit of the aminoacyl-tRNA synthetase complex is a parkin substrate: linking protein biosynthesis and neurodegeneration. Hum. Mol. Genet. 2003; 12: 1427–37.

137. Ren, Y., Zhao, J., Feng, J., Parkin binds to alpha/beta-tubulin and increases their ubiquination and degredation. J. Neurosci. 2003; 23: 3316–24.

138. Dong, Z., Ferger, B., Paterna, J.C., Vogel, D., Furler, S., et al. Dopamine-dependent neurodegeneration in rats induced by viral vector-mediated overexpression of the parkin target protein, CDCrel-1. Proc, Natl. Acad. Sci. USA. 2003; 100: 12438–43.

139. Murakami, T., Shoji, M., Imai, Y., Inoue, H., Kawarabayashi, T., et al. Pael-R is accumulated in Lewy bodies of Parkinson's disease. Ann. Neurol. 2004; 55: 439–42.

140. Wakabayashi, K., Engelender, S., Yoshimoto, M., Tsuji, S., Ross, C.A., Takahashi, H. Synphilin-1 is present in Lewy bodies in Parkinson's disease. Ann. Neurol. 2000; 47: 521–23.

141. Maraganore, D.M., Lesnick, T.G., Elbaz, A., Chartier-Harlin, M.C., Gaser, T., et al. UCHL1 is a Parkinson's disease susceptibility gene. Ann. Neurol. 2004; 55: 512–21.

142. Wilkinson, K.D., Lee, K.M., Deshpande, S., Duerksen-Hughes, P., Boss, J.M., Pohl, J., The neuron-specific protein PGP 9.5 is a ubiquitin carboxyl-terminal hydrolase. Science. 1989; 246: 670–73.

143. Lowe, J., McDermott, H., Landon, M., Mayer, R.J., Wilkinson, K.D. Ubiquitin carboxyl terminal hydrolase (PGP9.5) is selectively present in ubiquinated inclusion bodies chararacteristic of human neurodegenerative diseases. J. Pathol. 1990; 161: 153–60.

144. Liu, Y., Fallon, L., Lashuel, H.A., Liu, Z., Lansburg, P.T., Jr. The UCH-L1 gene encodes two opposing enzymatic activities that affect alpha-synuclein degradation and Parkinson's disease susceptibility. Cell. 2002; 111: 209–18.

145. Valente, E.M., Abou-Sleiman, P.M., Caputo, V., Musqit, M.M., Harvey K., et al, Hereditary early-onset Parkinson's disease caused by mutations in PINK1. Science. 2004; 304: 1158–60.

146. Bandopadhyay, R., Kingsbury, A.E., Cookson, M.R., Reid, A.R., Evans, I.M., et al. The expression of DJ-1 (PARK7) in normal human CNS and idiopathic Parkinson's disease. Brain. 2004; 127: 420–30.

147. Neumann, M., Muller, V., Gorner, K., Kretzschmar, H.A., Haass, C., Kahle, P.J. Pathological properties of the Parkinson's disease-associated protein DJ-1 in Alpha-synucleinopathies and tauopathies: relevance for multiple system system atrophy and Pick's disease. Acta. Neuropathol. (Berlin) 2004; 107: 489–96.

148. Rizzu, P., Hinkle, D.A., Zhukareva, V., Bonifati, V., Severijnen, L.A., et al. DJ-1 colocalizes with tau inclusions: a link between parkinsonism and dementia. Ann. Neurol. 2004; 55:113–18.

149. Moore, D.J., Zhang, L., Troncoso, J., Lee, M.K., Hattori, N., et al. Association of DJ-1 and perkin mediated by pathogenic DJ-1 mutations and oxidative stress. Hum. Mol. Genet. 2005; 14: 71–84.

150. Miller, D.W., Ahmad, R., Hague, S., Baptista, M.J., Canet-Aviles, R., et al. L166P mutant DJ-1, causative for recessive Parkinson's disease, is degraded through the ubiquitin-proteasome system. J. Biol. Chem. 2003; 278: n36588–95.

151. Moore, D.J., Zhang, L., Dawson, T.M., Dawson, V.L., A missense mutation (L166P) in DJ-1, linked to familial Parkinson's disease, confers reduced protein stability and impairs homo-oligomerization. J. Neurochem. 2003; 87: 1558–67.

152. Lee, S.J., Kim, S.J., Kim, I.K., Ko, J., Jeong, C.S., et al. Crystal structures of human DJ-1 and Escherichia doli Hsp31, which share an evolutionary conserved domain. J. Biol. Chem. 2003; 278: 44552–59.

153. Olzmann, J.A., Brown, K., Wilkinson, K.D., Rees, H.D., Huai, Q., et al. Familial

Parkinson's disease-associated L166P mutation disrupts DJ-1 protein folding and function. J. Biol. Chem. 2004; 279: 8506–15.

154. Taira,T., Saito, Y., Niki, T., Iguchi-Ariga, S.M., Takahashi, K., Ariga, H., DJ-1 has a role in antioxidative stress to prevent cell death. EMBO Rep. 2004; 5: 213–18.

155. Canet-Aviles, R.M., Wilson, M.A., Miller, D.W., Ahmad, R., McLendon, C., et al. The Parkinson's disease protein DJ-1 is neuroprotective due to cysteine-sulfinic acid-driven mitochondrial localization. Proc. Natl. Acad. Sci. USA. 2004; 101: 9103–8.

156. Yokota, T., Sugawara, K., Ito, K., Takahashi, R., Ariga, H., Mizusawa, H. Down regulation of DJ-1 enhancwes cell death by oxidative stress, ER stress, and proteasome inhibition. Biochem. Biophys. Res. Commun. 2003; 312: 1342–48.

157. Jenner, P. Oxidative stress in Parkinson's disease. Ann. Neurol. 2003; 53: S26–36.

158. Schapira, A.H., Cooper, J.M., Dexter, D., Clark, J.B., Jenner, P., Marsden, C.D. Mitochondrial complex 1 deficiency in Parkinson's disease. J. Neurochem. 1990; 54: 823–27.

159. Swerdlow, R.H., Parks, J.K., Miller, S.W., Tuttle, P.A., et al. Origin and functional consequences of the complex 1 defect in Parkinson's disease. Ann. Neurol. 1996; 40: 663–71.

160. Dauer, W., Prezsdborski, S. Parkinson's disease mechanisms and models. Neuron. 2003; 39: 889–909.

161. Tanaka, Y., Engelender, S., Igarashi, S., Rao, R.K., Wanner, T., et al. Inducible expression of mutant alpha-synuclein decreases propteasome activity and increases sensitivity to mitochondria-dependent apoptosis. Hum. Mol. Genet. 2001; 10: 919–26.

162. Chung, K.K., Thomas, B., Li, X., Plenikova, O., Troncoso, J.C., et al. S-nitrosylation of parkin regulates ubiniquination and compromises parkin's protective function. Science. 2004; 304: 1328–31.

163. Giasson, B.I., Lee, V.M. Are ubiquination pathways central to Parkinson's disease? Cell. 2003; 114: 1–8.

164. Moore, D.J., Dawson, V.L., Dawson, T.M. Role for the ubiquitin-proteasome system in Parkinson's disease and other neurodegenerative brain amyloidosis. Neuromolecular Med. 2003; 4: 95–108.

165. McNaught, K.S., Belizaire, R., Jenner, P., Olanow, C.W., Isacson, O. Selective loss od 20S proteasome alpha-subunits in the substancia nigra pars compacta in Parkinson's disease. Neurosci. Lett. 2002; 326: 155–58.

166. McNaught, K.S., Belizaire, R., Isacson, O., Jenner,P., Olanow, C.W. Altered proteasomal function in sporatic Parkinson's disease. Exp. Neurol. 2003; 179: 38–46.

167. Denovan-Wright, E.M., Rpbertson, H.A. Cannabinoid receptor messanger RNA levels decrease in subset neurons of the lateral striatum, cortex and hippocampus of transgenic Hungtington's disease mice. Neurosci. 2000; 98: 705–713.

168. Garcia-Arencibia, M., Garcia, C., Kurz, A., Rodriguez-Navarro, J.A., Gispert-Sachez, S., Mena, M.A., et al. Cannabinoid CB1 receptors and early downregulated followed by a further upregulation in the basal ganglia of mice with deletion of specific park genes. J. Neural. Transm. Suppl. 2009; 73: 269–75.

169. Ferrer, I., Martinez, A., Blanco, R., Dalfo, E., Carmona, M. Neuropathology of sporadic Parkinson's disease before the appearance of parkinsonism: preclinical Parkinson's disease. J. Neural. Transm. 2011; 118(5): 821–39. Doi: 10.1007/s00702-010-0482-8.

170. Garcia-Arencibia, M., Garcia, C., Fernandez-Ruis,J. Cannabinoids and Parkinson's disease, CNS Neurol. Disord. Drug Targets 2009; 8: 432–39.

171. Maccarone, M., Battista, N., Centonze, D. The endocannabinoid pathway in Huntington's disease: a comparison with other neurodegenerative diseases. Prog. Neurobiol. 2007; 81: 349–79.

172. Lastres-Becker, I., Molina-Holgado, F., Ramos, J.A., Mechoulam, R., Fernandez-Ruis, J. Cannabinoids provide neuroprotection against 6-hydroxydopamine toxicity in vivo and in vitro: relevance to Parkinson's disease. Neurobio. Dis, 2005; 19: 96–107.

173. Fernandez-Ruis, J., Moreno-Martet, M., Rodriguez-Cueto, C., Palomo-Garo, C., Gomez-Canas, M., et al. Prospects for cannabinoid therapies in basal ganglia disorders. Br. J. Pharmacol. 2011; 163: 1365–78.

174. Brotchie, J.M. CB1 receptor signaling in Parkinson's disease. Curr. Opin. Pharmacol. 2003; 3: 54–61.

175. Martin, A.B., Fernandez-Espejo, E., Ferrer, B., Gorriti, M.A., Bilbao, A., Navvaro, M., et al. Expression and function of CB1 receptor in the rat striatum: localization and effects on D1 and D2 dopamine receptor-mediated motor behaviors. Neuropsychopharmacology. 2008; 33: 1667–79.

176. Meschler, J.P., Howlett, A.C. Signal transduction interactions between CB1 cannabinoid and dopamine receptors in the rat and monkey striatum. Neuropharmacology. 2001; 40: 918–26.

177. Sanudo-Pena, M.C., Force, M., Tsou, K., Miller, A.S., Walker, J.M. Effects of intrastriatal cannabinoids on rotational behavior in rats: interactions with dopaminergic system. Synapse. 1998; 30:221–26.

178. Kreitzer, A.C., Malenka, R.C. Endocannabinoid-mediated rescue of striatal LTD and motor deficits in Parkinson's disease models. Nature. 2007; 445: 643–47.

179. Sagredo, O., Garcia-Arencibia, M., deLago, E., Finetti, S., Decio, A., Fernandez-Ruis, J. Cannabinoids and neuroprotection in basal ganglia disorders. Mol. Neurobiol. 2007; 36: 82–91.

180. Laciego, J.L., Barroso-Chiena, P., Rico, A.J., Conte-Perales, I., Callen, L., Roda, E., et al. Expression of the mRNA coding the cannabinoid receptor 2 in the pallidal complex of Macaca fasicularis. J. Psychopharmacol. 2011; 25: 97–104.

181. Fernandez-Ruis, J., Romero, J., Velasco, G., Tolon, R.M., Ramos, J.A., Guzman, M. Cannabinoid CB2 reeptor: a new target for controlling neural cell survival? Trends Pharmacol. Sci. 2007; 28: 39–45.

182. Fernandez-Ruis, J. The endocannabinoid system as a target for the treatment of motor dysfunction Br. J. Pharmacol. 2009; 156(7): 1029–40.

183. Fernandez-Ruis, J., Garcia, C., Sagredo, O., Gomez-Ruis, M., de Lago, E. The endocannabinoids system as a target for the treatment of neuronal damage. Expert. Opin. Ther. Targets. 2010; 14: 387–404.

HUNTINGTON'S DISEASE

1. Zuccato, C., Valenza, M., Cattaneo, E. Molecular mechanisms and potential therapeutic targets in Hungtion's disease. Physiol Rev. 2010,90: 905–81.

2. HD Collaborative Research Group. A novel gene containing a trinucleotide repeat that is expanded and unstable on Hungtington's disease chromosome. Cell. 1993; 72: 971–83.

3. Reiner, A., Albin, R.I., Anderson, K.D., D'Amato, C.J., Penny, J.B., Young, A.B. Differential loss of striatal projection neurons in Huntington's disease. Proc. Natl. Acad. Sci. USA. 1998; 85: 5733–37.

4. Rosas, H.D., Hevelone, N.D., Zaleta, A.K., Greve, D.N., Salat, D.H., Fischl, B. Regional cortical thinning in preclinical Huntington's disease and its relationship to cognition. Neurology. 2005; 65: 745–47.

5. Rosas, H.D., Koroshetz, W.J., Chen, Y.I., Skeuse, C., Vangel, M., Cudkowicz, M.E., et al. Evidence for more widespread cerebral pathology in early HD: an MRI-based morphometric analysis. Neurology. 2003; 60: 1615–20.

6. Rosas, H.D., Salat, D.H., Lee, S.Y., Zaleta, A.K., Pappu, V., Fischl, B., et al. Cerebral cortex and the clinical expression of Hungtington's disease: complexity and heterogeneity. Brain. 2008; 131: 1057–68.

7. Cattaneo, E., Zuccato, C., Tartari, M., Normal huntingtin function: an alternative approach to Hungtining's disease. Natl. Rev. Neurosci. 2005; 6: 919–30.

8. Zucatto, C., Cattaneo, E. Role of brain-deerived neurotrophic factor in Huntington's disease. Prog. Neurobiol. 2007; 81: 294–330.

9. Vonsattel, J.P., DiFiglia, M. Huntington's disease. J. Neuropathol. Exp. Neurol. 1998; 57: 369–84.

10. Kassubek, J., Juengling, F.D., Kioschies, T., Henkel, K., Karitzky, J., Kramer, B., et al. Topography of cerebral atrophy in early Huntington's disease: a voxel based morphometric MRI study. J. Neurol. Neurosurg. Psychiatry. 2004; 75: 213–20.

11. Politis, M., Pavese, N., Tai, Y.F., Tabrizi, S.J., Barker, R.A., Piccini, P. Hypothalamic involvement in Huntington's disease: an in vivo PET study. Brain. 2008; 131: 2860–69.

12. Bohanna, I., Georgiou-Karistianis, N., Hanman, A.J., Egan, G.F. Magnetic resonance imaging as an approach towards identifying neuropatholigical biomarkers for Huntington's disease. Brain Res. Rev. 2008; 58: 209–25.

13. Paulsen, J.S. Functional imaging in Huntington's disease. Exp. Neurol. 2009; 216:272–77.

14. Rosas, H.D., Feigin, A.S., Hersch, S.M. Using advances in neuroimaging to detect, understand and monitor disease progression in Huntington's disease. NeuroRx. 2004; 1: 263–72.

15. Rosas, H.D., Salat, D.H., Lee, S.Y., Zaleta, A.K., Hevelone, N., Hersch, S.M. Complexity and heterogenicity: what drives the ever-changing brain in Huntington's disease? Ann. NY Acad. Sci. 2008; 1147: 196–205.

16. Rosas, H.D., Tuch, D.S., Hevelone, N.D., Zaleta, A.K., Vangel, M., Hersch, S.M., Salat, D.H. Giffusion tensor imaging in presymptomatic and early Huntington's disease: selective white matter pathology and its relationship to clinical measures. Mov. Disord. 2006; 21: 1317–25.

17. Beighton, P., Hayden, M.R. Huntington's disease. S. Afr. Med.J. 1981; 59: 250

18. Conneally, P.M. Huntington's disease: genetics and epidemiology. Am. Hum. Genet. 1984; 36: 506–26.

19. Ashizawa, T., Wong, L.J., Richards, C.S., Caskey, C.T., Jankovic, J. CAG repeat size and clinical presentation in Huntington's disease. Neurology. 1994; 44: 1137–43.

20. Semaka, A., Collins, J.A., Hayden, M.R. Unstable familial transmission of Huntington's disease alleles with 27–35 CAG repeats (inter-mediate alleles) Am. J. Med. Genet.B. Neuropsychiatr Genet. 2010; 153: 314–20.

21. Andrew, S.E., Goldberg, Y.P., Kremer, B., Telenius, H., Theilmann, J., Adam, S., et al. The relationship between trinucleotide (CAG) repeat length and clinical features of Huntington's disease. Nat. Genet. 1993; 4: 398–403.

22. Rubinsztein, D.C., Barton, D.E., Davison, B.C., Ferguson-Sith, M.A. Analysis of the Huntington gene reveals a trinucleotide-length polymorphism in the region of the gene that contains two CCG-rich stretches and a correlation between decrease age of onset of Huntington's disease and CAG repeat number. Hum. Mol. Genet. 1993; 2: 1713–15.

23. Yamamoto, A., Lucas, J.J., Hen, R. Reversal of neuropathology and motor dysfunction in a conditional model of Huntington's disease. Cell. 2000; 101: 57–66.

24. Gu, X., Andre, V.M., Cepeda, C., Li, S.H., Li, X.J., Levine, M. S., Yang, X.W. Pathological cell-cell interactions are necessary for striatal pathogenesis in a conditional mouse model of Huntington's disease. Mol. Neurodegen. 2007; 2:8.

25. Harjes, P., Wanker, E.E. The hunt for huntingtin function: interaction partners tell many different stories. Trends. Biochem. Sci. 2003; 28: 425–33.

26. Atwal, R.S., Xia, J., Pinchev, D., Taylor, J., Epand, R.M., Truant, R., Huntingtin has a membrane association signal that can modulate huntingtin aggregation, nuclear entry and toxicity. Hum. Mol. Genet. 2007; 16: 2600–15.

27. Rockabrand, E., Slepko, N., Pantalone, A., Nukala, V.N., Kazantsev, A., Marsh, J.L., et al. The first 17-amino acids of Huntingtin modulate its sub-cellular localization, aggregation and effects on calcium homeostasis. Hum. Mol. Genet. 2007; 16: 61–77.

28. Fusco, F.R., Chen, Q., Lamoreaux, W.J., Figueredo-Cardenas, G., Jiao, Y., et al. Cellular localization of huntingtin in striatal and cortical neurons in rats: lack of correlation with neuronal vulnerability in Huntington's disease. J. Neurosci. 1999; 19: 1189–1202.

29. Hilditch-Maguire, P., Trettel, F., Passani, L.A., Auerbach, A., Persichetti, F., MacDonald,

M.E. Huntingtin: an iron-regulated protein essential for normal nuclear and perinuclear organelles. Hum. Mol. Genet. 2000; 9: 2789–97.

30. DiFiglia, M., Sapp, E., Chase, K., Schwarz, C., Young, C., Martin, E., et al. Huntingtin is a cytoplasmic protein with vesicles in human and rat brain neurons. 1995; 14: 1075–81.

31. Li, S.H., Li, X.J. Huntingtin-protein interactions and the pathogenesis of Huntington's disease. Trends. Genet. 2004; 20: 146–54.

32. Gauthier, L.R., Charrin, B.C., Borrell-Pages, M., Dompierre, J.P., Rangone, H., et al. Huntingtin controls neurotrophic support and survival of neurons by enhancing BDNF vesicular transport along microtubules. Cell. 2004; 118: 127–138.

33. Dietrich, P., Shanmugasundaram, R., Shuyu,E., Dragatsis, I. Congenital hydrocephalus associated with abnormal subcommissural organ in mice lacking huntingtin in Wnt1 cell lineages. Hum. Mol. Genet. 2009; 18: 142–50.

34. Gunawardena, S., Her, L.S., Brusch, R. G., Laymon, R.A., Niesman, I.R., et al. Disruption of axonal transport by loss of huntingtin or expression of pathogenic polyQ proteins in Drosophilia. Neuron 2003; 40: 25–40.

35. Smith, R., Brundin, P., Li, J.Y. Synaptic dysfunction in Huntington's disease: a new perspective. Ce.. Mol. Life. Sci. 2005; 62: 1901–12.

36. Reddy, P.H., Williams, M., Charles, V., Garrett, L., Pike-Buchanan, L., Whetsell, W.O. Jr., et al. Behavorial abnormalities and selective neuronal loss in HD transgenic mice expressing mutated full-length HD cDNA. Nat. Genet. 1998; 20: 198–202.

37. Leavitt, B.R., Guttman, J.A., Hodgson, J.G., Kimel, G.H., Singaraja, R., Vogl, A.W., Hayden, M.R. Wild-type huntingtin reduces the cellular toxicity of the mutant huntingtin in vivo. Am. J. Hum. Genet. 2001; 68: 313–24.

38. Zuccato, C., Tartari, M., Crotti, A., Goffredo, D., Valenza, M., Conti, I., et al. Huntingtin interacts with REST/NRSF to modulate the transcription of NRSE-controlled neuronal genes. Nat. Genet. 2003; 35: 76–83.

39. Altar, C.A., Cai, N., Bliven, T., Juhasz, M., Conner, J.M., Acheson, A.L., et al. Anterograde transport of brain-derived neurotrophic factor and its role in the brain. Nature. 1997; 389: 856–60.

40. Zucatto, C., Ciammola, A., Rigamonti, D., Leavitt, B.R., Goffredo, D., Conti, L., et al. Loss of huntingtin-mediated BDNF gene transcription in Huntington's disease. Science. 2001; 293: 493–8.

41. Ivkovic,S., Ehrlich, M.E. Expression of the striatal DARPP-32/ARPP-21 phenotype in GABAergic neurons requires neurotrophins in vivo and in vitro. J. Neurosci. 1999; 19: 5406–19.

42. Albin, R.I., Young, A.B., Penny, J.B., Handelin, B., Balfour, R., Anderson, K.D., et al. Abnormalities of striatal projection neurons and N-methyl-D-aspartate receptors in presymptomatic Huntington's disease. N. Engl. J. Med. 1990; 322: 1293–98.

43. Fan, M.M., Raymond, L.A. N-methyl-D-aspartate (NMDA) receptor function and excitotoxicity in Huntington's disease. Prog. Neurobio. 2007; 81: 272–93.

44. Cepeda, C., Wu, N., Andre, V.M., Cummings, C.M., Levine, M.S. The corticostriatal pathway in Huntington's disease. Prog. Neurobiol. 2007; 81: 253–71.

45. Sun, Y., Savanenin, A., Reddy, P.H., Lin, Y.F. Polyglutamine-expanded huntingtin promotes sensitization of N-methyl-D-aspartate receptors via post-synaptic density 95. J. Biol. Chem. 2001; 276: 24713–18.

46. Zeron, M.M., Fernandes, H.B., Krebs, C., Shehadeh, J., Wellington, C.L., Leavitt, B.R., et al. Potentiation of NMDA receptor-mediated excitotoxicity linked with intrinsic apoptotic pathway in YAC transgenic mouse model of Huntington's disease. MOL. CELL. NEUROSCI. 2004; 25: 469–79.

47. Choo, Y.S., Johnson, G.V., MacDonald, M., Detloff, P.J., Lesort, M. Mutant huntingtin directly increases susceptibility of mitochondria to the calcium-induced permeability transition and cytochrome c release. Hum. Mol. Genet. 2004; 13: 1407–20.

48. Bamford, N.S., Robinson, S., Palmiter, R.D., Joyce, J.A., Moore, C., Meshul, C.K. Dopamine modulates release from

corticostriatal terminals. J. Neurosci. 2004; 24: 9541–52.

49. Tarditi, A., Camurri, A., Varani, K., Borea, P.A., Woodman, B., Bates, G., et al. Early and transient alterations of adenosine A2A receptor signaling in a mouse model of Huntington's disease. Neurobiol. Dis. 2006; 23: 44–53.

50. Varani, K., Rigamonti, D., Sipione, S., Camurri, A., Borea, P.A., Cattabeni, F., et al. Aberant amplification of A2 receptor signaling in striatal cells expressing mutant huntingtin. FASB J. 2001; 15: 1245–47.

51. Maccarrone, M., Battista, N., Centonze, D, The endocannabinoid pathway in Huntington's disease: a comparison with other neurodegenerative diseases. Prog. Neurobiol. 2007; 81: 349–79.

52. Ona, V.O., Li, M., Vonsattel, J.P., Andrews, L.J., Khan, S.Q., Chung, W.M., Frey, A.S., et al. Inhibition of caspase-1 slows disease progression in a mouse model of Hungtington's disease. Nature. 1999; 399: 263–67.

53. Deng, Y., Slow, E.J., Haigh, B., Bissada, N., Lu, G., Pearson,J., Shehadeh, J., et al. Clevage at the caspase-6 site is required for neuronal dysfunction and degeneration due to mutant huntingtin. Cell. 2006; 125: 1179–91.

54. Bates, G. Hungtingtin aggregation and toxicity in Huntington's disease. Lancet. 2003; 361: 1642–44.

55. Ross, C.A. Huntington's disease new paths to pathogenesis. Cell. 2004; 118: 4–7.

56. Wanker, E.E. Protein aggregation and pathogenesis of Huntington's disease: mechanisms and correlations. Biol. Chem. 2000; 381: 937–42.

57. Thakur, A.K., Jayaraman, M., Mishra, R., Thakur, M., Chellgren, V.M., Byeon, I.J., et al. Polyglutamine disruption of the huntingtin exon 1 N terminus triggers a complex aggregation mechanism. Nat. Struct. Mol. Biol. 2009; 16: 380–9.

58. Hackam, A.S., Singaraja, R., Wellington, C.L., Metxler, M., McCutcheon, K., Zhang, T., et al. The influence of huntingtin protein size on nuclear localization and cellular toxicit. J, Ce.. Biol. 1998; 141: 1097–1105.

59. Ho, L.W., Brown, R., Maxwell, M., Wyttenbach, A., Rubinsztein, D.C. Wild type Huntingtin reduces the cellular toxicity of mutant Huntingtin in mammalian cell models of Huntington's disease. J. Med. Genet. 2001; 38: 450–52.

60. Yang, W., Dunlap, J.R., Andrews, R.B., Wetzel, R. Aggregated poly-glutamine peptides delivered to nuclei are toxic to mammalian cells. Hum. Mol. Genet. 2002; 11: 2905–17.

61. Cha, J.H. Transcriptional signatures in Huntington's disease. Prog. Neurobiol. 2007; 83: 228–48.

62. Nucifora, F.C., Jr., Ellerby, L.M., Wellington, C.L., Wood, J.D., Herring, W.J., Sawa, A., et al. Nuclear localization of a non-caspase truncation product of atrophin-1, with an expanded polyglutamine repeat, increases cellular toxicity. J. Biol. Chem. 2003; 278: 13047–55.

63. Bence, N.F., Sampat, R.M., Kopito, R.R. Impairment of the ubiquitin-proteasome system by protein aggregation. Science. 2001; 292: 1552–55.

64. DiFiglia, M., Sapp, E., Chase, K.O., Davies, S.W., Bates, G.P., Vonsattel, J.P., Aronin, n. Aggregates of huntingtin in neuronal intranuclear inclusions and dystrophic neuritis in brain. Science. 1997; 277: 1990–93.

65. Waelter, S., Boeddrich, A., Lurz, R., Scherzinger, E., Lueder, G., Lehrach, H., Wanker, E.E. Accumulation of mutant huntingtin fragments in aggresome-like inclusion bodies as a result of insufficient protein degredation. Mol. Biol>Cell. 2001; 12: 1393–1407.

66. Kuemmerle, S., Gutekunst, C.A., Klein, A.M., Li, X.J., Li, S.H., Beal, M.F., Hersch, S.M., Ferrante, R.J. Huntington aggregates may not predict neuronal death in Huntington's disease. Ann. Neurol. 1999; 46: 842–9.

67. Saudou, F., Finkbeiner, S., Devys, D., Greenberg, M.E. Huntingtin acts in the nucleus to induce apoptosis but death does not correlate with the formation of intranuclear inclusions. Cell 1998; 95: 55–66.

68. Ventruti, A., Cuervo, A.M. Autophagy and neurodegeneration .Curr. Neurol. Neurosci. Rep. 2007; 7: 443–51.

69. Ravikumar, B., Vacher, C., Berger, Z., Davies, J.E., Luo, S., Oroz, L.G., et al. Inhibition of mTOR induces autophagy and reduces toxicity of polyglutamine expansions in fly and mouse

models of Huntington's disease. Nat. Genet. 2004; 36: 585–95.

70. Orr, A.L., Li, S., Wang, C.E., Li, H., Wang, J., Rong, J., Xu, X., et al. NH-2 terminal mutant huntingtin associates with mitochondria and impairs mitochondrial trafficking. J. Neurosci. 2008; 28: 2783–92.

71. Panov, A. V., Burke, J.R., Strittmatter, W. J., Greenmyre, J.T. In vitro effects of polyglutamine tracts on Ca2+- dependent depolarization of rat and human mitochondria: relevance to Hungtington's disease. Arch. Biochem. Biophys. 2003; 410: 1–6

72. Browne, S.E., Ferrante, R.J., Beal, M.F. Oxidative stress in Huntington's disease. Brain Pathol. 1999; 9: 147–63.

73. Sipione, S., Rigamonti, D., Valenza, M., Zuccato, C., Conti, L., Pritchard, J., Kooperberg, C., et al. Early transcription profiles in huntingtin-induicible striatal cells by microarray analysis. Hum. Mol. Genet. 2002; 11: 1953–65.

74. Dietschy, J.M., Turley, S.D. Thematic review series: brain lipids. Cholesterol metabolism in the central nervous system during early development and in the mature animal. J. Lipid Res. 2004; 45: 1375–97.

75. Benn, C.L., Sun, T., Sadri-Vakilli, G., McFarland, K.N., DiRocco, D.P., Yohrling, G.J., Clark, T.W., Bouzou, B., Cha, J.H. Huntingtin modulates trtanscription, occupies gene promoters in vitro, binds directly to DNA in a polyglutamine-dependent manner. J. Neurosci. 2008; 28: 10720–33.

76. Sandri-Vakill, G., Bouzou, B., Benn, C.L., Kim, M.O., Chawla, P., Overland, R.P., et al. Histones associated with downregulated genes are hypo-acetylated in Huntington's disease models. Hum. Mol. Genet. 2007; 16: 1293–1306.

77. Fernandez-Ruis, J. The endocannabinoid system as a target for the treatment of motor dysfunction. Br. J. Pharmacol. 2009; 156(7): 1029–40.

78. Fernandez-Ruis, J., Gonzalez, S., Romero, J., Ramos, J.A. Cannabinoids in neurodegeneration and neuroprotection. In: Mechoulam, R. Ed., Cannabinoids as therapeutics (MDT), Birkhauser Verlag, Switzerland 2005; 79–109.

79. Fernandez-Ruis, J., Romero, J. Velasco, G., Tolon, R.M., Ramos, J.A., Guzman, M. Cannabinoid CB2receptor: a new target for the control of neural cell survival? Trends Pharmacol Sci. 2007; 28: 39–45.

80. Herkenham, M., Lynn, A.B., deCosta, B.R., Richfield, E.K. Neuronal localization of cannabinoid receptors in the basal ganglia of the rat. Brain Res. 1991; 547: 267–4.

81. Hohmann, A.G., Herkenham, M. Localization of cannabinoid CB1 receptor mRNA in neuronal subpopulations of rat striatum: a double-label in situ hybridization study synapse 2000; 37: 71–80

82. Pazos, M.R., Sagredo, O., Fernandez-Ruis, J. The Endocannabinoid system in Huntington's disease. Curr. Pharmacol. Design 2008; 14: 2317–25.

83. Sagredo, O., Garcia-Arencibia, M., deLago, E., Finetti, S., Decio, A., Fernandez-Ruis, J. Cannabinoids and neuroprotection in basal ganglia disorders. Mol Neurobiol. 2007; 36: 82–91.

84. Aiken, C.T., Tobin, A.J., Schweitzer, E.S. A cell-based screen for drugs to treat Huntington's disease. Neurobiol. Dis. 2004; 16: 546–55.

85. Wang, W., Duan, W., Igarashi, S., Morita, H., Nakamura, M., Ross, C.A. Compounds blocking mutant huntingtin toxicity identified using a Huntington's disease cell model. Neurobiol. Dis. 2005; 20: 500–8.

86. Lastres-Becker, E., Bizat, N., Boyer, F., Hantraye, P., Fernandez-Ruis, j., Brouillet, E. Potential involvement of cannabinoid receptors in 3-nitroproprionic acid toxicity in vivo. Neuroreport 2004; 15: 2375–9.

87. Sagredo, O., Ramos, J.A., Decico, A., Mechoulam, R., Fernandez-Ruis, J. Cannabidiol reduced the striatial atrophy caused by 3-nitropropionic acid in vivo by mechanisms independent of the activation of cannabinoid receptors. Eur. J. Neurosci. 2007; 26: 843–51.

88. Pintor, A., Tebano, M.T., Martire, A., Greico, R., Galluzzo, M., Scattoni, M.L. et al. The cannabinoid receptor agonist WIN 55,212–2 attenuates the effects induced by quinolinic

acid in the rat striatum. Neuropharmacoology 2006; 51: 1004–12.

89. Bonifati, D.M., Kishore, U. Role of complement in neurodegeneration and neuroinflammation. Mol Immuniol. 2007; 44: 999–1010.

90. Zhou, J., Bradford, H.F., Stern, G.M. Influence of BDNF on the expression of the dopaminergic phenotype of tissue used in brain transplants. Develop. Brain Res. 1997; 100: 43–51

91. Fernandez-Ruis, J., Sagredo, O., Pazos, M.R., Garcia, C., Pertwee, R., Mechoulam, R., Martinez-Orgado, J. Cannabidiol for neurodegenerative disorders: important new clinical applications for this phytocannabinoids. Br. J. Clin. Pharmacol. 2012; 75(2): 323–33.

92. Sagredo, O., Pazos, M.R., Satta, V., Ramos, J.A., Pertwee, R.G., Fernandez-Ruis, J. Neuroprotective effects of phytocannabinoids-based medicines in experimental models of Huntington's disease. J. Neurosci. Res. 2011; 89: 1509–18.

93. Valdeolivas, S., Satta, V., Pertwee, R.G., Fernandez-Ruis, J., Sagredo,O. Sativex-like combinations of phytocannabinoids is neuroprotective in malonate-lesioned rats, an inflammatory model of Huntington's disease: role of CB1 and CB2 receptors. ACS Chem. Neurosci. 2012; 3: 400–6.

94. Mechoulam, R., Parker, L.A., Gallily, R. Cannabidiol: an overview of some pharmacological aspects. J. Clin. Pharmacol. 2002; 42: 11S-9S.

95. Hampson, A.J., Grimaldi, M., Lolic, M., Wink, D., Rosenthal, R., Axelrod, J. Neuroprotective antioxidants from marijuana. N. Y. Acad. Sci. 2009; 899: 274–82.

96. El-Remessey, A.B., Kahill, I.E., Matragoon, S., Abou-Mohamed, G., Tsani, A.J., Roon, P., et al. Neuroprotective effect of (-) delta9-tetrahydrocannabinol and cannabidiol in N-methyl-D-aspartate-induced retinal neurotoxicity: involvement of peroxynitrite. Am. J. Pathol. 2003; 163: 1997–2008.

97. Hampson, A.J., Grimaldi, M., Axelrod, J., Wink, D., Cannabidiol and (-)delta9-tetrahydrocannabidiol are neuroprotective antioxidants. Proc, Natl. Acad. Sci. USA 1998; 95: 8268–73.

98. Marsicano, G., Moosman, B., Hermann, H., Lutz, B., Behl, C., Neuroprotective properties of cannabinoids against oxidative stress: role of cannabinoid receptor CB1. J. Neurochem. 2002; 80: 448–56.

99. Ruis-Valdepenas, L., Martinez-Orgado, J.A., Benito, C., Millam, A., Tolon, R.M., Romero, J. Cannabidiol reduces lipopolysaccharide-induced vascular changes and inflammation in the mouse brain: an intravital microscopy study. J. Neuroinflammation. 2011; 8: 5.

100. Martin-Moreno, A.M., Reigada, D., Ramirez, B.G., Mechoulam, R., Innamorato, N., Cuadrado, A., et al. Cannabidiol and other cannabinoids reduce microglial activation in vitro and in vivo: relevance to Alzheimer's disease. Mol Pharmacol. 2011; 79: 964–73.

101. Juknat, A., Pietr, M., Kozela, E., Rimmerman, N., Levy, R., Coppola, G., Geschwind, D., Vogel, Z. Differential transcriptional profiles mediated by exposure to the cannabinoids cannabidiol and delta9-tetrahydrocannabidiol in BV-2 microglial cells. Br. J. Pharmacol. 2012; 165: 2512–28.

102. Fernandez-Ruis, J. Garcia, C., Sagredo, O., Gomez-Ruis, M., deLago, E. The endocannabinoid system as a target for the tereatment of neuronal damage. Expert. Opin. Ther. Targets 2010; 14: 387–404

103. Walter, L., Franklin, A., Witting, A., Wade, C., Xie, Y., Kunos,G., Mackie, K., et al. Nonpsychotropic cannabinoid receptors regulat microglial cell migration. J. Neurosci. 2003; 23: 1398–405.

104. Esposito, G., Scuderi, C., Savani, C., Streado, L. Jr., DeFillips, D., Cottone, P., Iuvone, T., et al. Cannabidiol in vivo blunts beta-amyloid induced neuroinflammation by suppressing IL-1beta and iNOS expression. Br. J. Pharmacol. 2007; 151: 1272–9.

105. Esposito, G., DeFillips, D., Maiuri, M.C., DeStefano, D., Carnuccio, R., Iuvone, T. Cannabidiol inhibits inducible nitric oxide synthase protein expression and nitric oxide production in beta-amylooid stimulated PC12 neurons through p38MAP kinase and NF-kB involvement. Neurosci. Lett. 2006; 99: 91–5.

106. O'Sullivan, S.E., Kendall, D.A. Cannabinoid activation of peroxisome proliferator-activated receptors: potential for modulation od inflammatory disease. Immuniobuiology. 2010; 215: 611–6.

107. Esposito, G., Scuderi C., Valenza, M., Togna, G.I., Latina, V., DeFillips, D., et al. Cannabidiol reduces beta-amyloid-induced neuroinflammation and promotes hippocampal neurogenesis through PPARgamma involvement. Plos ONE. 2011; 6: e28668.

MULTIPLE SCLEROSIS

1. "Multiple Sclerorsis," Merck Manual, accessed August 29, 2015, http://www.merckmanuals.com/home/brain_spinal_cord_and_nerve_diso0rders/multiple_sclerosis_ms_and_related_disorders/multiple_sclerosis_ms.html.

2. "Multiple Sclerosis," Cleveland Clinic, accessed August 29, 2015, http:/www.clevlandclinicmeded.com/mediclpubs/diseasemanagement/neurology/multiple_sclerosis/

3. Cottrell, D.A., Kremenchutzky, M., Rice, G.P., et al. The natural history of multiple sclerosis: a geographically based study.5. The clinical features and natural history of primary progressive multiple sclerosis. Brain 1999; 122: 625–39.

4. Lucchinetti, C., Bruck, W., Parisi, J., Scheithauer, B., Rodriguez M., Lassman, H., Heterogenicity of multiple sclerosis lesions: implications for the pathogenesis of demyelination. Ann. Neurol. 2000; 47: 707–17.

5. Trapp, B.D., Peterson, J., Ransohoff, R.M., Rudick, R., Mork, S, Bo, L., Axonal transection in the lesions of multiple sclerosis. N. Engl. J. Med. 1998; 338: 278–85.

6. Lucchinetti, C.F., Propescu, B.F., Bunyan, R.F., et al. Inflammatory cortical demyelination in early multiple sclerosis. N. Engl. J. Med. 2011; 365: 2188–97.

7. Chang, A., Tourtellotte, W.W., Rudick, R., TrAPP, B.D. Premyelinating oligodendrocytes in chronic lesions of multiple sclerosis. N.ENGL. J. MED. 2002; 346: 165–73.

8. Schumacker, G.A. Beebe, G., Kibler, R.F., et al. Problems of experimental trials of therapy in multiple sclerosis: report by the panel on the evaluation of experimental trials of therapy in multiple sclerosis. Ann. N.Y. Acad. Sci. 1965; 122: 552–68.

9. McDonald, W.I., Compston, D.A., Edan, G., et al. Recommended diagnostic criteria for multiple sclerosis: guidelines from the International Panel on the diagnosis of multiple sclerosis. Ann. Neurol. 2001; 50: 121–27.

10. Fernandez-Ruis, J.J., Gonzalez, S., Romwro, J., Ramos, J.A. Cannabinoids in neurodegeneration and neuroprotection. Cannabinoids as Therapeutics. 2005. Birkhauser Verlag: Switzerland; 79–109. In; Mechoulam. R. (ed)

11. Glass, M. The role of Endocannabinoids in the Development, Progression, and Treatment of Neurodegenerative Diseases. Endocannabinoids The Brain and Body's Marijuana and Beyond. 2006 CRC Press, Boca Raton, Fla. 383–392. In: Onaivi, E., Sugiura, T., DiMarzo, V. (ed)

12. Arevalo-Martin, A., Vela, J.M., Molina-Holgado, E., Borrell, J., Gaza, C. Therapeutic action of cannabinoids in a murine model of multiple sclerosis. J. Neurosci. 2003; 23: 2511–16.

13. Caligano, A.G., LaRana, G., Giuffrida, A., Piomwlli, D. Control of pain initiation by endogenous cannabinoids. 1998; 394: 277–81.

14. Caligano, A., La Rana, G., Piomelli, D. Antinocioceptive activity of the endogenous fatty acid amide, palmitylethanolamide. Eur. J. Pharmacol. 2001; 419(2–3): 191–98.

15. Baker, D., Pryce, G., Croxford, J.L., Brown, P., Pertwee, R.G., Huffman, J.W., Layward, L. Cannabinoids control spasticity and tremor in Multiple sclerosis model. Nature. 2000; 404(6773): 84–7.

16. Baker, D., Pryce, G., Croxford, J.L., Brown, P., Pertwee, R.G., Makriyannis, A., Khanolka, A., Layward, L., et al. Endocannabinoids control spasticity in a multiple sclerosis model. FASEB J. 2001; 15(2): 300–2.

17. Molina-Holgado, F., Molina-Holgado, E., Guaza, C. The endogenous cannabinoid anandamide potentiates interleukin-6 production by astrocytes infected with Theiler's murine encephalomyelitis virus by a

receptor-mediated pathway. FEBS. Lett. 1998; 433(1–2): 139–42.

18. Booz, G.W. Cannabidiol as an emergent therapeutic strategy for lessening the impact of inflammation on oxidative stress. Free Radic. Biol. Med. 2011; 51(5): 1054–61.

19. Carrier, E.J., Auchampach, J.A., Hillard, C.J. Inhibition of an equilibrative nucleoside transporter by cannabidiol: a mechanism of cannabinoid immunosuppression. Proc. Natl. Acad, Sci. USA. 2006; 103:7895–7900.

20. Kozela, E., Pietr, M., Juknat, A., Rimmerman, N., Levy,R., Vogel, Z. Cannabinoids delta-9-tetrahydrocannabinol and cannabidiol differentially inhibit the lip[osaccahride-activated NF-k and interferon-Beta/STAT proinflammatory pathways in BV-2 microglial cells. J. Biol. Chem. 2010; 285: 1616–26.

21. Kim, D., You, B., Jo, E.K., Simon, M.I., Lee, S.J. NADPH oxidase2-derived reactive oxygen species in spinal cord microglia contribute to peripheral nerve injury-induced neuropathic pain. Proc. Natl. Acad. Sci. USA. 2010; 107: 14851–56.

22. Toth, C.C., Jedrzejewski, N.M., Ellis, C.L., Frey, W.H. 2nd Cannabinoid-mediated modulation of neuropathic pain and microglial accumulation in a mouse of murine type 1 diabetic neuropathic pain. Mol. Pain 2010; 6:16.

23. Mecha, M., Feliu, A., Inigo, P.M., Mestre, L., Carillo-Salinas, F.J., Guaza, C. Cannabidiol provides long-lasting protection against deleterious effects of inflammation in a viral model of multiple sclerosis: A role for A2A reeptors. Neurobiol. Dis. 2013; 59: 141–50.

24. Archelos, J.J., Previtali, S.C., Hartung, H.P. The role of intergins in immune-mediated diseases of the nervous system. Trends. Neurosci. 1999; 22: 30–38.

25. Rajesh, M., Mukhopadhyay, P., Butkai, S., Hasko, G., Liaudet, L., Huffman, J.W., Csiszar, a., et al. CB2-receptor stimulation attenuates TNF-alpha-induced human endothelial cell activation, transendothelial migration of monocytes, and monocyte-endothelial adhesion. Am. J. Physiol. Heart Circ. Physiol. 2007; 293: H2210-H2218.

26. Glass, W.G., Rosenberg, H.F., Murphy, P.M. Chemokine regulation of inflammation during acute viral infection. Curr. Opin. Allergy Clin. Immuniol. 2003; 3: 467–73.

27. Hoffman, L.M., Fife, B.T., Begolka, W.S., Miller, S.D., Karpus, W.J. Cental nervous system chemokine expression during Theiler's virus-induced demyelinating diseaqse. J. Neurovirol. 1999; 5: 635–42.

28. Tanasescu, R., Constantinescu, C.S. Cannabinoid and the immune system: an overview. Immunobiol. 2010; 215: 588–97.

29. Kozela, E., Lev, N., Kaushansky, N., Eilam, R., Rimmerman, N., Levy, R., Ben-Nun, A., et al. Cannabidiol inhibits pathogenic T cells, decreases spinal microglial activation and ameliorates mjltiple sclerosis-like disease in C57BL6 mice. Br. J. Pharmacol. 2011; 163(7): 1507–19.

30. Mecha, M., Torrao, A.S., Mestre, L., Carrillo-Salinas, F.J., Mechoulam, R., Guaza, C. Cannabidiol protects oligodendrocytes progenitor cells from inflammation-induced a poptosis by attenuating endoplasmic reticulum stress. Cell Death and Disease. 2012; 3, e331; doi: 10.1038/eddis.2012.71.

31. Levine, J.M., Reynolds, R., Fawcett, J.W. The oligodendrocytes precursor cell in health and disease. Trends Neurosci. 2001; 24: 39–47.

32. Stetka, B. Could Multiple Sclerosis begin in the gut? Scientific American. Oct. 8, 2014.

PAIN

1. Cravatt,B.F., Lichtman,, A.H. The endogenous cannabinoid system and its role in nocioceptive behavior. J. Neurobiol. 2004; 98: 149–160.

2. Hohmann, A.G., Suplita, R.L. II. Endocannabinoid mechanisms of pain modulation. AAPS J 2006; 8: E693–708.

3. Jhaveri, M.D., Richardson, D., Chapman, V. Endocannabinoid metabolism and uptake: novel targets for neuropathic and inflammatory pain. Br, J. Pharmacol. 2007; 152: 634–52.

4. Walker, J.M., Krey, J.F., Chu, C.J., Huang, S.M. Endocannabinoids and related fatty acid deravitives in pain modulation. Chem Phys Lipids. 2002; 121:159–72.

5. Kano, M., Ohno-Shosaku, T., Hashimotodani, Y., Uchigashima, M., Watanabe, M. Endocannabinoid-mediated control of synaptic Transmission. Physiol. Rev. 2009; 89: 309–80.

6. Hohmann, A.G., Suplita, R.L., Bolton, N.M., Neely, M.H., Fegley, D., et al. An endocannabinoid mechanism for stress-induced analgesia, Nature. 2005; 435: 1108–1112.

7. Ashton, J.C., Milligan, E.D. Cannabinoids for the treatment of neuropathic pain: clinical evidence. Curr. Opin. Invest. Drugs. 2008; 9: 65–75.

8. Rog, D.J., Nurmikko, T.J., Friede, T., Young, C.A. Randomized, controlled trial of cannabis-based medicine in central pain in multiple sclerosis. Neurology. 2005; 65:812–819.

9. Snyder, S.H. (1971) Uses of Marijuana, Oxford University Press, New York.

10. Zias, J., Stark, H., Sellgman, J., Levy, R., Werker, E., Breuer, A., Mechoulam, R. Early medical use of cannabis. Nature. 1993; 363; 215.

11. Hohmann, A.G., Martin, W.J., Tsou, K., Walker, J.M. Inhibition of noxious stimulus-evoked activity of spinal cord dorsal horn neurons by the cannabinoid WIN 55,212. Life Sci. 1995; 56: 2111–2118.

12. Hohmann, A.G., Tsou, K., Walker, J.M. Cannabinoid modulation .of wide dynamic range neurons in the lumbar dorsal horn of the rat by spinnaly administered WIN 55,212. Neurosci. Lett. 1998; 257: 119–122.

13. Hohmann, A.G., Tsou, K., Walker, J.M. Cannabinoid suppression of noxious heat-evoked activity in a wide dynamic range of neurons in the lumbar dorsal horn of the rat. J. Neurophys. 1999; 81: 575–583.

14. Martin, W.J., Hohmann, A.G., Walker, J.M. Suppression of noxious stimulus-evoked activity in the ventral posteriolateral nucleus of the thalamus by a cannabinoid agonist: correlation between electrophysical and antinociceptive effects. J. Neurosci. 1996; 16: 6601–6611.

15. Strangman, N.M., Walker, J.M. The cannabinoid WIN 55,212-2 inhibits the activity-dependent facilitation of spinal nocioceptive responses. J. Neurophys. 1999; 81: 472–477.

16. Martin, W.J., Coffin, P.O., Attias, E., Balinsky, M., Tsou, K., Walker, J.M. Anatomical basis for cannabinoid-induced antinocioception as revealed by intracerebral microinjections. Brain Res. 1999; 822: 237–242.

17. Martin, W.J., Patrick, S.L., Coffin, P.O., Tsou, K., Walker, J.M. An examination of the central sites of action of cannabinoid induced antinocioception in the rat. Life Sci. 1995; 56: 2103–2109.

18. Martin, W.J., Tsou, K., Walker, J.M. Cannabinoid receptor-mediated inhibition of the rat tail-flick reflex after microinjection into the rostral ventromedial medulla. Neurosci. Lett. 1998; 242: 33–36.

19. Lichtman, A.H., Martin, B.R. Cannabinoid induced antinocioception is mediated by a spinal alpha2-noradrenergic mechanism. Brain. Res. 1991; 559: 309–314.

20. Gutierrez, T., Nackley, A.G., Neeley, M.H., Freeman, K.G., Edwards, G.L., Hohmann, A.g. Effects of neurotoxic destruction of descending noradrenergic pathways on cannabinoid antinocioception in models of acut and tonic nocioception. Brain Res. 2003; 987: 176–185.

21. Gilbert, P.E. A comparison of THC, nantradol, nabilone and morphine in the chronic spinal dog. J. Clin. Pharmacol. 1981; 21: 311S-319S.

22. Kelly, S., Chapman, V. Selective cannabinoid CB 1 receptor activation inhibits spinal nocioceptive transmission in vivo. J. Neurophysiol. 2001; 86: 3061–3064.

23. Richardson, J.D., Kilo, S., Hargreaves, K.M. Cannabinoids reduce hyperalgesia and inflammation via interaction with peripheral CB1 receptors. Pain. 1998; 75: 111–119.

24. Huang, S.M., Walker, J.M. Cannabinoid targets for pain therapies. Cannabinoids as Therapeutics. 2005. Birkhauser Verlag: Switzerland; 149–164. In; Mechoulam, R. (ed.)

25. Malan, T.P. Jr., Ibrahim, M.M., Deng, H., Liu,Q., Mata, H.P., et al. CB2 cannabinoid receptor-mediated peripheral antinocioception. Pain. 2001; 93: 239–245.

26. Clayton, N., Marshall, F.H., Bountra, C., O'Shaughnessy, C.T. CB1 and CB2

cannabinoid receptors are implicated in inflammatory pain. Pain. 2002; 96: 253–260.

27. Hanus, L., Breuer, A., Tchilibon, S., Shiloah, S., Goldenberg, D., et al. HU-308: A specific agonist for CB(2), a peripheral cannabinoid receptor. Proc. Natl. Acad. Sci. USA. 1999; 96: 14228–14233.

28. Hohmann, A.G., Farthing, J.N., Zvonok, A.M., Makriyannis, A. Selective activation of cannabinoid CB2 receptors suppresses hyperalgesia evoked by intradermal capsaicin. J. Pharmacol. Exp. Ther. 2004; 308: 446–453.

29. Ibrahim, M.M., Deng, H., Zvonok, A., Cockayne, D.A., Kwan, H.P., et al. Activation of CB2 cannabinoid receptors by AM1241 inhibits experimental neuropathic pain: Pain inhibition by receptors not present in the CNS. Proc. Natl. Acad. Sci USA. 2003; 100: 10529–10533.

30. Griffin, G., Fernando, S.R., Ross, R.A., McKay, N.G., Ashford, M.L., et al. Evidence for the presence of CB2-like cannabinoid receptors on peripheral nerve terminals. Eur. J. Pharmacol. 1997; 339: 53–61.

31. Zeidenberg, P., Clark, W.C., Jaffe, J., Anderson, S.W., Chin, S., Malitz, S. Effect of oral administration of delta-9-tetrahydrocannabinol on memory, speech, and perception of thermal stimulation: results with four normal human volunteer subjects. Preliminary Report. Compr. Psychiatry. 1973; 14: 549–556.

32. Raft, D., Gregg,J., Ghia, J., Harris, L. Effects of intravenous tetrahydrocannabinol on experimental and surgical pain. Psychological correlates of the analgesic response. Clin. Pharmacol. Ther. 1977; 21: 26–33.

33. Noyes, R. Jr., Brunk, S.F., Avery, D.A., Canter, A.C. The analgesic properties of delta-9-tetrahydrocannabinol and codeine. Clin. Pharmacol. Ther. 1975; 18: 84–89.

34. Noyes, R. Jr., Brunk, S.F., Baram, D.A., Cantar, A. Analgesic effect of delta-9-tetrahydrocannabinol. J. Clin. Pharmacol. 1975; 15: 139–143.

35. Kehl, L.J., Hamamoto, D.T., Wacnik, P.W., Croft, D.L., Norsted, B.D., Wilcox, G.L., Simone, D.A. A cannabinoid agonist differentially attenuates deep tissue hyperalgesia

in animal model of cancer and inflammatory pain. Pain 2003; 103: 175–186.

36. Svendsen, K.B., Jensen, T.S., Bach, F.W. Does the cannabinoid dronabinol reduce central pain in multiple sclerosis? Randomised double blind placebo controlled trial. Br. Med. J. 2004; 329: 253.

37. Prather, P.L., Martin, N.A., Breivogel, C.S., Childers, S.R. Activation of cannabinoid receptors in rat brain by WIN 55212–2 produces coupling to multiple G protein alpha-subunits with different potencies. Mol Pharmacol. 2000; 57: 1000–1010.

38. Houston, D.B., Howlett, A.C. Differential receptor-G-protein coupling evolked by dissimilar cannabinoid receptor agonists. Cell Signal. 1998; 10: 667–674.

39. Glass, M., Northup, J.K. Agonist selective regulation of G proteins by cannabinoid CB(1) and CB(2) receptors. Mol. Pharmacol. 1999; 56: 1362–1369.

40. Mukhopaddhyay, S., Howlett, A.C. CB1 receptor G-protein association. Subtype selectivity is determined by distinct intracellular domains. Eur. J. Biochem. 2001; 268: 499–505.

41. Romero, J., Lastres-Becker, I., de Miguel, R., Berrendero, F., Ramos, J.A., Fernandez-Ruis, J.J. The endogenous cannabinoid system and the basal ganglia.biochemical, pharmacological and therapeutic aspects. Pharmacol. Ther. 2002; 95: 137–152.

42. Walker, J.M., Hohmann, A.G., Martin, W.J., Stangman, N.M., Huang, S.M., Tsou, K. The neurobiology of cannabinoid analgesia. Life Sci. 1999; 65: 665–673.

43. Hohmann, A.G. Spinal and peripheral mechanisms of cannabinoid antinocioception: behavioral, neurophysiological and neuroanatomical perspectives. Chem. Phys. Lipids. 2002; 121: 173–190.

44. DiMarzo, V., Bisogno, T., Sugiura, T., Melck, D., DePetrocellis, L. The novel endogenous cannabinoid 2-arachidonylglycerol is inactivated by neuronal- and basophil-like cells: connections with anandamide. Biochem. J. 1998; 331: 15–19.

45. Huang, S.M., Bisogno, T., Trevisani, M., Al-Haymani, A., DePertocellis, L., Fezza, F., et

al. An endopgenous capsaicin-like substance with high potency at recombinant and native vallinoid VR1 receptors. Proc. Natl. Acad. Sci. USA. 2002; 99: 8400–8405.

46. Cravatt, B.F., Demarest, K., Patricelli, M.P., Bracey, M.H., Giang, D.K., et al. Supersensitivity to anandamide and enhanced endogenous cannabinoid signaling in mice lacking fatty acid amide hydrolase. Proc. Natl. Acad. Sci. USA. 2001; 98: 9371–9376.

47. Beltramo, M., Stella, N., Calignano, A., Lin, S.Y., Makriyannis, A., Pimonelli, D. Functional role of high-affinity anandamide transport, as revealed by selective inhibition Science. 1997; 277: 1094–1097.

48. Manzanares, J., Julian, M.D., Carrascosa,A. Role of the cannabinoid System in pain control and therapeutic implications for the management of acute and chronic pain episodes. Curr. Neuropharmacol. 2006; 4(3): 239–257.

49. Lichtman A.H., Cook, S.A., Martin, B.R. Investigation of brain sites mediating cannabinoid-induced antinocioception in rats, evidence supporting periaqueductal gray involvement. J. Pharmacol. Exp. Ther. 1996; 276: 585–593.

50. Ibrahim, M.M., Porreca, F., Lai, J., Albrecht, P.J., Rice, L., et al. CB2 cannabinoid receptor activation produces antinocioception by stimulating peripheral release of endogenous opioids. Proc. Natl. Acad. Sci. USA. 2005; 102: 3093–3098.

51. Fowler, C.J. Possible involvement of the endocannabinoid system in the actions of three clinically used drugs. Trends. Pharmacol Sci. 2004; 25: 59–61.

52. Holt, S., Fowler, C.J. Anandamide metabolism by fatty acid amide hydrol; ase in intact C6 glioma cells. Increased sensitivity to inhibition by ibuprofen and flurbuprofen upon reduction of extra- but not intracellular pH. Naunyn Schmiedeberg Arch Pharmacol. 2003; 367: 237–244.

53. Gopez, J.J., Yue, H., Vasudevan, R., Malik, A.S., Fogelsanger, L.N., et al. Functional outcomes, provides neu-roprotection, and reduces inflammation in a rat model of tramatic brain injury. Neurosurgery. 2005; 56: 590–604.

54. Mao, J., Price, D.D., Lu, J., Keniston, L., Mayer, D.J. Two distinctive antinocioceptive systems in rats with pathologic pain. Neurosci. Lett. 2000; 280: 13–16.

55. Pryce, G., hmed, Z., Hankey, D.J., Jackson, S.J., Croxford, J.L., et al. Cannabinoids inhibit neu-rodegeneration in models of multiple sclerosis. Brain. 2003; 126: 2191–2202.

56. Hohmann, A.G., Herkenham, M. Localization of central cannabinoid CB1 receptor messanger RNA in neuronal subpopulations of rat dorsal root ganglia, a double label in situ hybridization study. Neuroscience. 1999; 90: 923–931.

57. Radbruch, L., Elsner, F. Emerging analgesics in cancer pain management. Expert Opin. Emerg. Drugs. 2005; 10: 151–171.

58. Russo, E. Cannabis for migraine treatment: the once and future prescription? An historical and scientific review. Pain. 1998; 76: 3–8.

59. Noyes, R., Jr., Baram, D.A. Cannabis analgesia. Compr. Psychiatry. 1974; 15: 531–535.

60. Toth, C.C., Jedrzejewski, N.M., Ellis, C.L., Frey, W.H. Cannabinoid-mediated modulation of neuropathic pain and microglial accumulation in a model of murine typeI diabetic peripheral neuropathic pain. Molecular Pain. 2010; 6: 16. doi 10.1186/1744–8069-6–16.

61. Xiong,W., Cui, T., Cheng, K., Yang, F., Chen, S.R., et al. Cannabinoids suppress inflammatory and neuropathic pain by targeting alpha-3 glycine receptors. J Exper. Med. 2012; 209(6): 1121–1134. Doi: 10.1084/jem.20120242.

62. Abrams, D.I., Couey,P., Shade, S.B., Kelly, M.E., Benowitz, N.L. Cannabinoid-Opioid interaction in chronic pain. Clinic. Pharmacol. Ther. 2011; 90(6): 844–51. doi:10.1038/clpt.2011.188.

63. Nackley, A.G., Zvonok, A.M., Makriyannis, A., Hohmann, A.G. Activation of cannabinoid CB2 receptors suppress spinal fos protein expression and pain behavior in a rat model of inflammation. Neuroscience. 2003; 119: 747–757.

64. Portenoy, R.K., Ganae-Motan, E.D., Allende, S., Yanagihara, R., Shaiova, L., et al. Nabiximols for opioid-treated cancer patients with poorly-controlled pain: a randomized,

placebo-controlled, graded dose trial. J. Pain. 2012; 13(5): 438–49. Doi: 10.1016/j. pain.2012.01.003.

65. Beltramo,M., Bernardin, N., Bertorelli, R., et al. Cb2 receptor mediatedantihyperalgesia: possible direct involvement of neural mechanisms. Eur. J. Neurosci. 2006; 23: 1530–1538.

66. Wotherspoon, G., Fox, A., McIntyre, P., Colley, S., Bevan, S., Winteer, J. Peripheral nerve injury induces cannabinoid receptor 2 protein expression in rat sensory neurons. Neuroscience 2005; 135: 235–245.

67. Guindon, J., Hohmann, A.G. Cannabinoid CB 2 receptors: a therapeutic target for the treatment of inflammatory and neuropathic pain. Br. J. Pharmacol. 2008; 153: 319–34.

68. Rahn, E.J., Hohmann, A.G. Cannabinoids as pharmacotherapies for neuropathic pain: from the bench to the bedside. Neurotherapeutics. 2009; 6(4): 713–37.

69. Mechoulam, R., Peters, M., Murillo-Rodriguez, E., Hanus, L.O. Cannabidiol-recent advances. Chem. Biodivers 2007; 4: 1678–92.

70. Racz, ., Alfernink, J., et al. Interferon-gamma is a critical modulator of CB (2) cannabinoid receptor signaling during neuropathic pain. J. Neurosci. 2008; 28: 12136–45.

71. Zhang, F., Hong, S., Stone, V., Smith, P.J. Expression of cannabinoid CB1 receptors in models of diabetic neuropathy. J. Pharmacol. Exp. Ther. 2007; 323: 508–15.

72. Matias, I., Wang, J.W., Moriello, A.S., Nieves, A., Woodward, D.F., Di Marzo, V. Changes in endocannabinoid levels in eye tissues with diabetic retinaopathy and age related macular degeneration. Prostaglandins leukot. Essent Fatty Acids. 2006; 75: 413–18.

73. Olechowski, C.J., Troung, J.J., Kerr, B.J. Neuropathic pain behaviors in a chronic-relapsing model of experimental autoimmune encephalomyelitis. (E.A.E.) Pain. 2009; 141: 156–64.

74. Racz, I., Nadal, X., Alfrerick, J., Banos, J.E., Rehnelt, J., Martin, M., et al. Crucial role of CB2 Cannabinoid receptor in the regulation of

central immune responses during neuropathic pain. J. Neurosci. 2008; 28(46): 12125–12135.

75. Yang, K.H., Galadari, S., Isaev, D., Petroianu, G., Shippenberg, T.S., Oz, M. The nonpsychoactive cannabinoid cannabidiol inhibits Hydroxytryptamine-3a receptor-mediated currents in Xenopus laevis oocytes. J. Pharmacol. Exper. Ther. 2010; 333: 547–54.

NAUSEA AND VOMITING

1. Parker, L.A. Limebeer, C.L., Kwiatkowska, M. Cannabinoids: effects on vomiting and nausea in animal models. Cannabinoids as Therapeutics. 2005. Birkhauser Verlag: Switzerland; 183–200. In; Mechoulam, R. (ed.)

2. Andrews, P_.L.R., Davis, C.J. The physiology of emesis induced by anti-cancer therapy. In: J. Reynolds, Andrews, P.L.R., Davis, C.J. (eds): Serotonin and the scientific basis of anti-emetic therapy. Oxford Clinical Communications, Oxford, 25–49.

3. Slatkin, N.E. Cannabinoids in the treatment of chemotherapy-induced nausea and vomiting: Beyond prevention of acute emesis. J. Support Oncology. 2007; 5(Supp3): 1–9.

4. Costall, B., Domeney, A.M., Naylor, R.J., Tattersal, F.D. 5-Hydroxytryptamine receptor antagonism to prevent cisplatinum-induced emesis. Neuropharmacol. 1986; 25: 959–961.

5. Matusiak, N., Ueno, S., Kaji, T., Ishihara, A., Wang, C.H., Saito, H. Emesis induced by cancer chemotherapeutic agents in the Suncus murinus: A new experimental model. Jpn. Pharmacol. 1998; 48: 303–306.

6. Miner, W.J., Sanger, G.J. Inhibition of cisplatinum-induced vomiting by selective 5-hydroxytryptamine a-receptor antagonism. Br. J. Pharmacol. 1986; 88: 497–499.

7. Torii,Y., Saito, H., Matuski, N. Selective blockade of cytotoxic-induced emesis by 5-HT3 receptor antagonist in Suncus murinus. Japan J. Pharmacol. 1991; 55: 107–113.

8. Ueno, S., Matsuki, N., Saito, H. Suncus murinus: A new experimental model in emesis research. Life Sci. 1987; 43: 513–518.

9. Aapro, M.S., Thuerlimann, B., Sessa, C., DePree, C., Bernhard, J., Maibach,R.;

Swiss group for Clinical Cancer research, A randomized double-blind trial compare the clinical efficacy of grainstron with metoclopramide, both combined with dexamethasone in the prophylaxis of chemotherapy-induced delayed emesis. Ann. Occolo. 2003; 14: 291–297.

10. Barlett, N., Koczwara, B. Control of nausea and vomiting after chemotherapy; what is the evidence? Int.Med.J. 2002; 32: 401–407.

11. Hickock, J.T., Roscoe, J.A., Morrow, G.R., King, D.K., Atkins, J.N., Fitch, T.R. Nausia and emesis remain significant problems of chemotherapy despite prophylaxis with 5-Hydroxytramine-3 antiemetics. Cancer. 2003; 97: 2880–2886.

12. Schnell, F.M. Chemotherapy-induced nausea and vomiting: The importance of acute antiemetic control. Oncologist. 2003; 8: 187–198.

13. Reynolds, D.J.M., Barber, N.A., Grahame-Smith, D.G., Leslie, R.A. Cisplatinum-evoked induction of c-fos protein in the brainstem of the ferrit: The effect of cervical vagotomy and the antiemetic 5HT-3 receptor antagonist graisetron. Brain Res. 1991; 565: 321–336.

14. Tsukada, H., Hirose, T., Yokoyama, A., Kurita,Y. Randomizied comparison of ondansetron plus dexamethasone with dexamethasone alone for control of delayed cisplatinum-induced emesis. Eur. J. Cancer. 2001; 37: 2398–2404.

15. Ballatori, E., Roila, F. Impact of nausea and vomiting on quality of life in cancer patients during chemotherapy. Health Qal. Life Outcomes 2003; 1:46

16. Parker, L.A., Rock, E.M., Limebeer, C.L. Regulation of nausea and vomiting by cannabinoids. Br.J. Pharmacology. 2011; 163(7): 1411–22. Br, J. Pharmacol.-Wiley online library Http://onlinelibrary.wiley.com/doi/10.1111/j.1476–5381.2010.01176.x/full.

17. Sanger, G.J., Andrews, P.L. Treatment of nausea and vomiting: gaps in our knowledge. AutonNeurosci. 2006; 129: 3–16.

18. Hornby, P.J. Central neurocircuitry associated with emesis. Am. J. Med. 2001; 111(suppl 8A): 106S-112S.

19. Van Sickle, M.D., Oland, H.O., Hillard, C.J., Mackie, K., Davison, J.S., et al. Cannabinoid: inhibit emesis through CB1 receptors in the brainstem of the ferret. Gastroenterology 2001; 121: 767–74.

20. Daramini, N.A., McClanahan, B.A., Trinh, C., Petrosino, S., Valenti, M., DiMarzo, V. Cisplatinum increases brain 2-arachidonylglycerol (2-AG) and concomitantly reduces intestinal 2-AG and anandamide levels in the least shrew. Neuropharmacology. 2005; 49: 502–13.

21. Van Sickle, M.D., Oland, L.D., Ho, W., Hillard, C.J., Mackie, K., Davison, J.S., et al. Cannabinoid: inhibit emesis through CB1 receptors in the brainstem of the ferret. Gastroenterology. 2001; 121: 767–74.

22. Van Sickle, M.D., Oland, L.D., Mackie, K., Davison, J.S., Sharkey, K.A. delta-9-tetrahydrocannabinol selectively acts on CB1 receptors in specific regions of the dorsal vagal complex to inhibit emesis in ferrets. Am. J. Physiol. Gastrointest. Liver Physiol. 2003; 285: G566-G576.

23. Darmani, N.A., Johnson, C.J. Central and peripheral mechanisms contribute to the antiemetic actions of delta-9-tetrahydrocannabinol against 5-hydroxytryptophan-induced emesis. Eur. J. Pharmacol. 2004; 488: 201–12.

24. Van Sickle, M.D., Cuncan, M., Kingsley, P.J., Mouihate, A., Urbani, P., Mackie, K., et al. Identification and functional characterization of brainstem cannabinoid CB2 receptors. Science. 2005; 213: 329–32.

25. Sharkey, K.A., Cristino, L., Oland, L.D., Van Sickle, M.D., Starowicz, K., Pittman, Q.J., et al. Arvanil, anandamide and N-arachidonoyl-dopamine (NADA) inhibited emesis through CB1 and Vanilloid TRPV1 receptors in the ferret. Eur. J. Neurosci. 2007; 25: 2773–82.

26. DiMarzo, V., Fontana, A. Anandamide, an endogenous cannabinomimetic eicosanoid: 'killing two birds with one stone'. Prostaglandins Leukot. Essent. Fatty Acids. 1995; 53: 1–11.

27. Kimura, T., Ohta, T., Watanabe, K., Yoshimura, H., Yamamoto, I. Anandamide, an endogenous cannabinoid receptor ligand, also interacts with 5-hydroxytryptamine (5HT) receptor. Biol. Pharm. Bull. 1998; 21: 224–26.

28. Himmi, T., Dallaporta, M., Perrin, J., Orsini, J.C. Neuronal responses to delta-9-tetrahydrocannabinol in the solitary tract nucleus. Eur. J. Pharmacol. 1996; 312: 273–79.

29. Himmi, T., Perrin,J., ElOuazzani, T., Orsini, J.C. Neuronal responses to cannabinoid receptor ligands in the solitary tract nucleus. Eur. J. Pharmacol. 1998; 359: 49–54.

30. Fan, P. Cannabinoid agonist inhibit the activation of 5-HT3 receptors in rat nodose ganglion neurons. J. Neurophysiol. 1995; 73: 907–10.

31. Barann, M., Molderings, G., Bruss, M., Bonisch, H., Urban, B.W., Gothert, M. Direct inhibition by cannabinoids of human 5-HT-3A receptors: probable involvement of an allosteric modulatory site. Br. J. Pharmacol. 2002; 137: 589–96.

32. Mechoulam, R., Parker, L.A., Gallily R. Cannabidiol: an overview of some pharmacological aspects. J. Clin. Pharmacol. 2002; 42: 11S-19S.

33. Kwiatkowski, M., Parker, L.A., Burton, P., Mechoulam, R. A comparative analysis of the potential of cannabinoids and ondansetron to suppress cisplatinum-induced emesis in the Suncus murinus (house musk shrew). Psychopharamcology 2004; 174: 254–59.

34. Parker, L.A., Kwiatkowska, M., Burton, P., Mechoulam, R. Effect of cannabinoids on Lithium-induced vomiting in the Suncus murinus. Psychopharmacology 2004; 171: 156–61.

35. Parker, L.A., Kwiatkowska, M., Mechoulam, R. Delta-9-tetrahydrocannabinol and cannabidiol, but not ondanstron, interfere with conditioned retching reactions elicited by a lithium-paired context in Suncus murinus: an animal model of anticipatory nausea and vomiting. Physiol. Behav. 2006; 87: 61–71.

36. Pertwee, R.G. The Pharmacology and Therapeutic Potential of Cannabidiol. DiMarzo, V. (ed.) Kluver Academic/Plenum Publishers: Cannabinoids.

37. Darmani, N.A. The potent emetogenic effects on the endocannabinoid, 2-AG(2-arachidonoylglycerol) are blocked by delta-9-tetrahydrocannibinol and other cannabinoids. J. Pharmacol. Exp. Ther. 2002; 300: 34–42.

38. Russo, E.B., Burnett, A., Hall, B., Parker, K.K. Agonist properties of cannabidiol at 5-HT1A receptors. Neurochem. Res. 2005; 30: 1037–43.

39. Blier, P., de Montigny, C. Modification of 5-HT neuron properties by sustained administration of the 5-HT1A agonist gepirone: electrophysiological studies in the rat brain. Synapse 1987; 1: 470–80.

40. Yang, K.H., Galadari, S., Isaev, D., Petroianu, G., Shippenberg, T.S. The nonpsychoactive cannabinoid cannabidiol inhibits 5-Hydroxytryptamine 3A receptor-mediated currents in Xenopus laevis Oocytes. J. Pharmacol. Exp. Ther. 2010; 333: 547–54.

41. Andrews, P.L., Horn, C.C. Signals for nausea and emesis: implications for models disease. Auton Neurosci. 2006; 125: 100–15.

42. Reynolds, D.J.M., Barber, N.A., Grahame-Smith, D.G., Leslie, R.A. Cisplatin-evoked induction of c-fos protein in the brainstem of the ferret: the effect of cervical vagotomy and the antiemetic 5HT-3 receptor antagonist granistron. Brain Res. 1991; 565: 321–36.

43. Travers, J.B., Norgen, R. Electromyeographic analysis of the ingestion and rejection of sapid stimuli in the rat. Behav. Neurosci. 1986; 100: 544–55.

44. Limebeer, C.L., Parker, L.A. Delta-9-tetrahydrocannabinol interfers with the establishment and the expression of conditioned disgust reactions by cyclophosphamide: a rat model of nausea Neuroreport. 1999; 26: 371–84.

45. Parker, L.A., Mechoulam, R. Cannabinoid agonist and antagonist modulate conditioned gaping in rats. Integr. Physiol. Behav. Sci. 2003; 38: 134–46.

46. Parker, L.A., MechoulamR., Shlievert, C., Abbott, L., Fudge, M.L., Burton,P. Effects of cannabinoids on lithium-induced conditioned rejection reactions in a rat model of nausea. Psychopharmacology. 2003; 166: 156–62.

47. Cross-Mellor, S.K., Ossenkopp, K.P., Piomelli,D., Parker, L.A. Effects of the FAAH inhibitor, URB597, and anandamide on lithium-induced taste reactivity response: a measure of nausea in the rat. Psychopharmacology 2007; 190: 135–43.

48. Tuerke, K.J., Limebeer, C.L., Lester, J., Chambers, J., Fletcher, P.J., Parker, L.A. Depletion of serotonin in the insular cortex by 5,67-Dihydroxytrptamine (5,7-DHT) lesions attenuates conditioned nausea in rats. J. Neurosci. 2012; 32(40): 13709–17.

49. Nesse, R.M., Carli, G.C., Kleinman, P.D. Pretreatment nausea in cancer chemotherapy: a conditioned response? Psychosom. Med. 1980; 42: 33–36.

50. Pavlov, I.P. Conditioned Reflexes. (G.V. anrep, trans.). Oxford University Press: London, England.

51. Rock, E.M., Limebeer, C.L., Mechoulam, R., Piomelli, D., Parker, L.A. The effect of cannabidiol and URB597 on conditioned gaping (a model of nausea) elicited by a lithium-paired context in the rat. Psychopharmacology 2008; 196: 389–395.

ARTHRITIS

1. Osteoarthritis, Stedmans Medical Dictionary, 27th Ed; Lippincott Williams & Wilkins, Baltimore MD., USA

2. Berenbaum, F. Osteoarthritis as an inflammatory disease (osteoarthritis is not osteoarthrosis!). Osteoarthritis and Cartilage. 2013; 21(1): 16–21. doi:10:1016/j.joa.2012.11.012

3. Conaghan, P., "Osteoarthritis - National Clinical Guideline for Care and Management in Adults", National Institute for Health and Care Excellence, Feb 2008, http://www.nice.org.uk/nicemedia/pdf/cg059FullGuideline.pdf.

4. Centers for Disease Control and Prevention (CDC) Prevalence of disabilities and associated health conditions among adults—United States, 1999.(FEB. 2001), MMWR Morb. Mortal. Wkly. Rep. 50(7): 120–5.

5. VanManen, M.D., Nace, J., Mont, M.A. Management of primary knee osteoarthritis and indications for total knee arthroplasty for general practitioners. J. Am. Osteopath. Assoc. 2012; 112(11): 709–15.

6. Shah, Ankur. Harrison's Principles of Internal Medicine (18th ed.). United States: McGraw Hill.. p. 2738.

7. Majithia, V., Geraci, S.A, Rheumatoid arthritis: diagnosis and management. Am. J. Med. 2007; 120(11): 936–9.

8. Nicki, R.C., Brian, R.W., Stuart, HR., ed. (2010). Davidson's Principles and Practice of Medicine. (21st ed.) Edinburgh: Churchill Livingstone/Elserve.

9. Dunn, S.L., Wilkinson, J.M., Crawford, A., Le Maitre, C.L., Bunning, R.A. Cannabinoids: novel therapies for arthritis? Future Med. Chem. 2012; 4(6):713–25. doi:10.4155/fmc.12.20.

10. Mbvundula, E.C., Bunning, R.A., Rainsford, K.D. Arthritis and cannabinoids: HU-210 and WIN-55,212,2 prevent IL-1alpha induced matrix degredation in bovine articular chondrocytes in-vitro. J. Pharm. Pharmacol. 2006; 58(3): 351–8.

11. Malfait, A.M., allily, R., Sumariwalla, P.F., Malik, A.S., Andreakos, E., Mechoulam, R., Feldmann, M. The non-psychotropic cannabis constituent cannabidiol is an oral anti-arthritic therapeutic in murine collagen-induced arthritis. Proc. Natl. Acad. Sciences. 2000; 97(17): 9561–66. Doi: 10.1073/pnas.160105897.

12. Booz, G.W. Cannabidiol as an emergent therapeutic strategy for lessening the impact of inflammation on oxidative stress. Free Rad. Biol. & Med. 2011; 51; 1054–61.

13. McHugh, D., Tanner, C., Mechoulam, R., Pertwee, R.G., Ross, R.A. Inhibition of human neutrophil chemotaxis by endogenous cannabinoids and phytocannabinoids: evidence for a site distinct from CB1 and CB2. Mol. Pharmacol. 2008; 73: 441–50.

14. ElRemessy, A.B., Tang, Y., Zhu, G., Matragoon, S., Khalifa, Y. et al. Neuroprotective effects of cannabidiol in endotoxin-induced uveitis: critical role of p38 MAPK activation. Mol. Vis. 208; 14: 2190–2203.

15. Mechoulam, R., Peters, M., Murillo-Rodriguez, E., Hanus, L.O. Cannabidiol-Recent Advances. Chem. Biodivers. 2007; 4: 1678–92.

16. Gowran, A., McKayed, K., Kanichai, M., White, C., Hammadi, N., Campbell, V. Tissue Engineering of cartilage; Can Cannabidiol Help? Pharmaceuticals 2010; 3: 2970–85. Doi:10.3390/ph3092970.

17. Whyte, L.S., Ryberg, E., Sims, N.A., Ridge, S.A., Mackie, K., Greasley, P.J. et al. The putative cannabinoid receptor GPR55 affects osteoclast function in vitro and bone mass in vivo. aProc. Natl. Acad Sci. USA. 2009; 106: 16511–16.

18. Stebulis, J.A., Johnson, D.R., Rossetti, R.G., Burnstein, S.H., Zurier, R.B. Ajulemic acid, a synthetic cannabinoid acid, induces an anti-inflammatory profile of eicosanoids in human synovial cells. Life Sci. 2008; 83: 666–70.

19. Burstein, S.H. Ajulemic acid (CT3): a potent analogue of the acid metabolites of THC. Curr. Pharm. Des. 2000; 6: 1339–45.

20. Zurier, R.B., Sun, Y.P., George, K.L., Stebulis, J.A., Rossetti, R.G., et al. Ajulemic acid, a synthetic cannabinoid, increases formation of the endogenous proresolving and anti-inflammatiory eicosanoid, lipoxin A4. FASEB J. 2009; 23: 1503–09.

21. McPartland, J.M., Skinner, E. The biodynamic model of osteopathy in the cranial field. Explore (NY) 2005; 1: 21–32.

22. Blake, D.R., Robson,P., Ho, M., Judd, R.W., McCabe, C.S. Preliminary assessment of the efficacy, tolerability and safety of a cannabis-based medicine (Sativex) in the treatment of pain caused by rheumatoid arthritis. Rheumatology. 2006; 45(1): 50–52.

23. Selvi, E., Lorenzini, S., Garcia-Gonzalez, ., Maggio, R., Lazzerini, P.E., Capecchi, P.L., et al. Inhibitory effect of synthetic cannabinoids on cytokine production in rheumatoid fibroblast-like synovicytes. Clin. Experim. Enviro. Rheumatology 2008:26:574–81.

24. Fukuda, S., Kohsaka, H., Takayasu, A., Yokoyama, W., Miyabe,C., et al. Cannabinoid receptor2 as a potential therapeutic target in rheumatoid arthritis. BMC Musculosketal Disord. 2014; 15: 275–83. Doi: 10.1186/1471-2474-15-275.

25. Richardson, D., Pearson, R.G., Kurian, N., Latif, M.L., Garle, M.J., Barrett, D.A., et al. Chacterization of the cannabinoid receptopr system in synovial tissue and fluid in patients wit osteoarthritis and rheumatoid arthritis. Arthritis Res. Ther. 2008; 10(2): R43. Doi:10.1186/ar2401.

26. Ofek, O., Karsak, M., Leclerc, N., Fogel,M., Frenkel, B., Wright, K., et al. Peripheral cannabinoid receptor, CB2, regulates bone mass. Proc. Natl.Acad. Sci. USA. 2006; 103: 696–701. Doi:10.1073/pnas.0504187103.

27. Mechoulam, R., Fride, E., DiMarzo, V. Endocannabinoids. Eur. J. Pharmacol. 1998; 359: 1–18. Doi: 10.1016/S0014-2999(98)00649-9.

28. Lambert, D.M., DiMarzo, V. The palmitoylethanolamide and oleamide enigmas: are these two fatty acis amides cannabimimetic? Curr. Med. Chem. 1999; 6: 757–73.

29. Lambert, D.M., Vandevoorde, S., Jonsson, K.O., Fowler, C.J. The palmitoyletanolamide family: a new class of anti-inflammatory agents? Curr. Med. Chem. 2002; 9: 663–74.

30. Baker, C.L., McDougal, J.J. The cannabinometric arachidonyl-2-chloroethylamide (ACEA) acts on capsaicin sensitive TRPV1 receptors but not cannabinoid receptors in rat joints. Br. J. Pharmacol. 2004; 142: 1361–67.

31. Kimball, E.S., Schneider, C.R., Wallace, N.H., Hornby, P.J. Agonist of cannabinoid receptor 1 and 2 inhibit experimental colitis induced by oil of mustard and by dextran sulfate sodium. Am.J. Physiol. Gastrointes. Liver Physiol.2006; 291: G364-G371.

32. McDougall, J.J., Yu, V., Thomson, J. In vivo effects of CB2 receptor- selective cannabinoids on the vasculature of normal and arthritic rat knee joints. Br. J. Pharmacol. 2008; 153(2): 358–66.

33. Shoemaker, J.L., Joseph, B.K., Ruckle, M.B., Mayeux, P.R., Prather, P.L. The endocannabinoid noladin ether acts as a full agonist at human CB2 receptors. J. Pharmacol. Ther. 2005; 314: 868–75.

34. Fan, T., Tao, Q., Abood, M., Martin, B.R. Cannabinoid receptor down-regulation without alteration of the inhibitory effect of CP55940 on adenyl cyclase in the cerebellum of CP55940-tolerant mice. Brain. Res. 1996; 706: 13–20.

CANCER

1. Mellors, R.C., "Etiology of Cancer : Carcinogenesis, Neoplasia," Med Path, 2006, http://www.medpath.info/Main Content/Neoplasia/Neoplasia_04.html.

2. "Epigenetic therapy", Nova, Oct 16, 2007, http://www.pbs.org/wgbh/nova/body/epigenetic-therapy.html.

3. Pisani, P., Bray, F., Parkin, D.M. Estimates of the world-wide prevalence of cancer for 25 sites in the adult population. Int. J. Cancer. 2002; 97: 72–81. Doi: 10.1002/ijc.1571.

4. Parolaro, D., Massi, P. Cannabinoids as potential new therapy for the treatment of gliomas. Exp. Rev. Neurotherapies. 2008; 8(1): 37–49.

5. Bouaboula, M., Poinot-Chazel, C., Bourrie, B., et al. Activation of mitogen-activated protein kinase by stimulation of the central cannabinoid receptor CB1. Biochem. J. 1995; 312: 637–41.

6. Rueda, D., Galve-Roperth, I., Haro, A., Guzman, M., The CB(1) cannabinoid receptor is coupled to the activation of c-Jun N-Terminal kinase. Mol. Pharmacol. 2000; 58: 814–20.

7. Liu, J., Gao, B., Mirshahi, F., et al. Functional CB1 cannabinoid receptors in human vascular endothelial cells. Biochem. J. 2000; 15: 835–40.

8. Gomez del Pulgar, T., De Ceballos, M., Guzman, M., Velasco, G. Cannabinoids protect astrocytes from ceramide-induced apoptosis through the phosphatidylinositol 3-kinase/protein kinase B pathway. L. Biol. Chem. 2002; 39: 36527–36533.

9. Derkinderen, P., Toutant, M., Burgaya, F., et al. Regulation of a neuronal form of focal adhesion kinase by anandamide. Science. 1996; 273: 1719–22.

10. Gomez del Pulgar, T., Velasco, G., Sanchez, C., Haro, A., Guzman, M. De novo-synthesized ceramide is involved in cannabinoid-induced apoptosis. Biochem.J. 2002; 363: 183–88.

11. Sathornsumetee, S., Reardon, D., Dejardins, A., Quinn, J.A., Verdenburgh, J.J., Rich, J.N. Molecularly targeted therapy for malignant glioma. Cancer 2007; 110: 13–24.

12. Sanchez,C., Galve-Roperh, I., Canova, C., Brachet, P., Guzman, M. Delta-9-tetrahydrocannabinol induces apoptosis in C6 glioma cells. FEBS Lett. 1998; 436: 6–10.

13. Galve-Roperth, I., Sanchez, C., Cortes, M.L., et al. Anti-tumorial action of cannabinoids: involvement of sustained ceramide accumulation and extracellular signal-regulated kinase activation. Nat. Med. 2000; 6: 313–19.

14. Guzman, M., Galve-Roperth, I., Sanchez, C. Ceramide: a new second messenger of cannabinoid action. Trends. Pharmacol. Sci. 2001; 22: 19–22.

15. Carracedo, A., Geelen, M.J., Diez, M., Hanada, K., Guzman, M., Velasco, G. Ceramide sensitizes astrocytes to oxidative stress: protective role of cannabinoids. Biochem. J. 2004; 380: 435–40.

16. Carracedo, A., Lorente, M., Egia, A., et al. The stress-regulated protein p8 mediates cannabinoid-induced apoptosis of tumor cells. Cancer Cell. 2006; 9: 301–12.

17. Guzman, M., Sanchez, C., Galve-Roperth, I. Cannabinoids and cell fate. Phasrmacol. Ther. 2002; 95: 175–84.

18. Massi, P., Vaccani, A., Bianchessi, S., Costa, B., Macchi, P., Parolaro, D. The non-psychoactive cannabidiol triggers caspase activation and oxidative stress in human glioma cells. Cell. Mol. Life Sci. 2006; 63: 2057–66.

19. Sanchez, C., de Ceballos, M.L., del Pulgar, T.G., et al. Inhibition of glioma growth in vivo by selective activation of the CB(2) cannabinoid receptor. Cancer Res. 2001; 61: 5784–89.

20. Massi,P., Vaccani,A., Ceruti, S., Colombo, A., Abbracchio, M.P., Parolaro, D. Antitumor effects of cannabidiol, a nonpsychoactive cannabinoid, on human glioma cell lines. J. Pharmacol. Exp. Ther. 2004; 308: 838–45.

21. Riboni, L., Campanella, R., Bassi, R., et al. Ceramide levels are inversely associated with malignant progression of human glial tumors, Glia. 2002; 39: 105–113.

22. Ellert-Miklaszewska, A., Kaminska, B., Konarska, L. Cannabinoids down-regulate P13K/Akt and ERK signaling pathways and activate proapoptotic functions of Bad protein. Cell. Signal. 2005; 17: 25–37.

23. Blazquez, C., Gonzales-Feria, L., Alvarez, L., Haro, L., Llanos Casanova, M., Guzman, M. Cannabinoids inhibit the vasacular endothelial growth factor pathway in gliomas. Cancer. Res. 2004; 64: 5617–23.

24. Blazquez,C., Casanova, M.L., Planas, A., et al. Inhibition of tumor angiogenesis by cannabinoids. FASEB J. 2003; 17: 529–31.

25. Vaccani, A., Massi, P., Colombo, A., Rubino, T., Parolaro, D. Cannabidiol inhibits human glioma cell migration through a cannabinoid receptor-independent mechanism. Br. J. Pharmacol. 2005; 144: 1032–1036.

26. Blazquez, C., Carracedo, A., Salazar, M., et al. Down-regulation of tissue inhibitor of metalloproteinase-1 in gliomas: a new marker of cannabinoid antitumoral activity? Neuropharmacol. 2008; 54(1): 235–43.

27. Sekhon, B.S. Matrix metalloproteinases- an Overview. Res. And Reports in Biology. 2010; 1:1–20.

28. Blazquez, c., Casanova, M.L., Planas, A., Del Pulgar, T.G., Villanueva, C., et al. Inhibition of tumor angiogenesis by cannabinoids. FASEB J. 2003; 17(3): 529–31.

29. Solinas, M., Massi, P., Cantelmo, A.R., Cattaneo, M.G., Cammarota, R., et al. Cannabidiol inhibits angiogenesis by multiple mechanisms. Br. J. Pharmacol. 2012; 167(6): 1218–31.

30. Blazquez, C., Salazar,M., Carracedo, A., Lorente, M., Egla, A., et al. Cannabinoids inhibit Glioma cell invasion by down-regulating Matrix Metalloproteinase-2 Expression. Cancer Res. 2008; 68: 1945–52.

31. Blazquez, C., Gonzalez-Feria, L., Alvarez, L., et al. Cannabinoids inhibit the vascular endothelial growth factor pathway in Gliomas. Cancer Res. 2004; 64:5617–23.

32. Guzman, M. Cannabinoids: potential anticancer agents. Nat. Rev. Cancer. 2003; 3:745–55.

33. Massi,P., Solinas, M., Cinquina, V., Parolaro, D. Cannabidiol as potential anticancer drug. Br. J. Clin. Pharmacol. 2012; 75: 303–12.

34. Howlett, A>C. The cannabinoid receptors. Prostaglandins. Other lipid Mediat. 2002; 68–69: 619–31.

35. Van Sickle, M.D., Duncan, M., Kingsley, P.J., Mouihate, A., Urbani, P., Mackie, K., et al. Identification and functional characterization of brainstem cannabinoid CB2 receptors. Science. 2005; 310: 329–32.

36. Ross,R.A. Anandamide and Vanilloid TRPV1 receptors. Br. J. Pharmacol. 2003; 140: 790–801.

37. Ryberg, E., Larsson, N., Sjogren, S., Hjorth, S., Hermansson, N.O., et al. The orphan receptor GPR 55 is a novel cannabinoid receptor. Br. J. Pharmacol. 2007; 152: 1092–101.

38. O'Sullivan, S.E. Cannabinoids go nuclear: evidence for activation of peroxisomal proliferator-activated receptors. Br. J. Pharmacol. 2007; 152: 576–82.

39. Pertwee, R.G., Howlett, A.C., Abood, M.E., Alexander, S.P., DiMarzo, V., et al. International Union of Basic and Clinical Pharmacology. LXXIX. Cannabinoid receptors and their ligands: beyond CB1 and CB2. Pharmacol. Rev. 2010; 62: 588–631.

40. Freimuth, an., Ramer, R., Hinz, B. Antitumorigenic effects of cannabinoids beyond apoptosis. J. Pharmacol, Exp. Ther. 2010; 332: 236–44.

41. Massi, P., Vaccani, A., Ceruti, S., Colombo, A., Abbracchio, M.P., Parolaro, D. Antitumor effects of cannabidiol, a nonpsychoactive cannabinoid, on human glioma cell lines. J. Pharmacol. Exp. Ther. 2004; 308: 838–45.

42. McAllister, S.D., Murase, R., Christian, R.T., Lau, D., Zielinski, A.J., et al. Pathways mediating the effects of cannabidiol on the reduction of breast cancer cell proliferation, invasion and metastasis. Breast Cancer Res. Treat. 2011; 129: 37–47.

43. Shrivastava, A., Kuzontkoski, P.M., Groopman, J.E., Prasada, A. Cannabidiol induces programmed cell death in breast cancer cells by coordinating the cross-talk between apoptosis and autophagy. Mol. CANCER THER. 2011; 10: 1161–72.

44. Jacobsson, S.O., Rongard, E., Stridh, M., Tiger, G., Fowler, C.J. Serum-dependent effects of tamoxifen and cannabinoids upon C6 glioma cell viability. Biochem. Pharmacol. 2000; 60: 1807–13.

45. Valenti, M., Massi, P., Bolognini, D., Solinas, M., Parolaro, D. Cannabidiol, a non-psychoactive cannabinoid compound, inhibits human glioma cell migration and invasiveness. 34th National Congress of the Italian Society of Pharmacology 2009.

46. Marcu, J.P., Christian, R.T., Lau, D., Zielinski, A.J., Horowitz, M.P., et al. Cannabidiol enhances the inhibitory effects of delta-9-tetrahydrocannabinol on human glioblastoma cell proliferation and survival. Mol. Cancer Ther. 2010; 9: 180–9.

47. Massi, P., Valenti, M., Vacani, A., Gasperi, V., Perletti, G., Marras, E., et al. 5-Lipoxygenase and anandamide hydrolase (FAAH) mediated the antitumor activity of cannabidiol, a non-psychoactive cannabinoid. J. Neurochem. 2008; 104: 1091–100.

48. Ligresti, A., Moriello, A.S., Starowicz, K., Matias, I., Pisanti, S., et al.Antitumor activity of plant cannabinoids with emphasis on the effects of cannabidiol on human breast carcinoma. J. Pharmacol. Exp. Ther. 2006; 318: 1375–87.

49. McAllister, S.D., Christian, R.T., Horowitz, M.P., Garcia, A., Desprez, P.Y. Cannabidiol as a novel inhibitor of Id-1 gene expression in aggressive breast cancer cells. Mol. Cancer Ther. 2007; 6: 2921–7.

50. Cho, D.H., Jo, Y.K., Hwang, J.J., Lee, Y.M., Roh, S.A., Kim, J.C. Caspase-mediated cleavage of ATG6/Beclin-1 links apoptosis to autophagy in HeLa cells. Cancer Lett. 2009; 274: 95–100.

51. Wirawan, E., Vande Walle, L., Kersse, K., Cornelis, S., Claerhout, S., Vanoverberghe, I., et al. Caspase-mediated cleavage of Beclin-1 inactivates Beclin-1 induced autophagy and enhances apoptosis by promoting the release of proapoptotic factors from mitochondria. Cell Death Dis. 2010; 1: e18.

52. McKallip, R.J., Jia, W., Schlomer, J., Warren, J.W., Nagarkatti, P.S., Nagarkatti, M. Cannabidiol induced apoptosis in human leukemia cells: a novel role of cannabidiol in the regulation of p22phox and NOX4 expression. Mol. Pharmacol. 2006; 70: 897–908.

53. McKallip, R.J., Lombard, C., Fisher, M., Martin, B.R., Ryu, S., Grant, S., et al Targeting CB2 cannabinoid receptors as a novel therapy to treat malignant lymphoblastic disease. Blood. 2002; 100: 627–34.

54. Ramer, R., Merkord, J., Rohde, H., Hinz, B. Cannabidiol inhibits cancer cell invasion via upregulation of tissue inhibitor of matrix metalloproteinase-1. Biochem. Pharmacol 2010; 79: 955–66.

55. Ramer, R., Merkord, J., Rohde,H., Hinz, B. Decrease of plasminogen activator inhibitor-1 may contribute to the anti-invasive action of cannabidiol on human lung cancer cells. Pharm. Res. 2010; 27: 2162–74.

56. Ramer, R., Hinz, B. Inhibition of cancer cell invasion by cannabinoids via increased expression of tissue inhibitor of matrix metalloproteinase-1. J. Natl. Cancer Inst. 2008; 100: 59–69.

57. Aviello, G., Romano, B., Borrelli, F., Capasso, R., Gallo, L., Piscitelli, F., et al. Chemoprotective effect of the non-psychotropic phytocannabinoids cannabidiol on experimental colon cancer. J. Mol. Med. (Berl) 2012; 90(8): 925–34.

58. Rieder, S.A., Chauhan, A., Singh, U., Nagarkatti, M., Nagarkatti, P. Cannabinoid-induced apoptosis in immune cells as a pathway to immunosuppression. Immuniobiology. 2010; 215: 598–605.

Glossary

Acetylcholine—an acetic ester of choline, used by some neurons as a neurotransmitter.

Adenylate cyclase/ adenylyl cyclase—the activity of this compound is inhibited by the stimulation of cannabinoid receptors, this leads to their activity and responses in the cells when these receptors are used.

Adjuvant—an additional therapy to enhance or extend the primary therapies effects.

Afferent nocioceptors—a peripheral nerve organ which transmit information to the brain about pain or injury.

Agonism—a compound that stimulates a receptor and produces a reaction, such as stimulating a drug receptor and causing the same reaction.

Akt/mTOR/4EBP1—this is a signaling pathway that helps regulate the cell cycle, this is used by cancer cells to aide survival, when it is blocked the cells loose ability to adjust and control their survival.

Alpha-synuclein—a protein that is found at the ends of neurons, function not fully understood, in Parkinson's disease it is seen to fold and therefore cannot be removed or broken down; it is believed to be involved in dopamine release and uptake.

Analgesia—reduction of pain.

Antagonism—opposition in action to structures, agents, physiologic processes, neutralize, create a different or block the action of an agonist.

Antigens—cell surface markers which are specific to each cell, they can induce a state of sensitivity and/or immune responsiveness.

Anxiolytic—an action or compound to reduce anxiety.

Astrocytes—one type of glial or supportive neuroglial cells.

Autophagy—consumption of a cell from its own digestive components.

Basophils—a granulocyte with basic staining granules, in blood and tissues, contains inflammation activating substances.

Beclin 2—a protein associated with cell death from autophage, it is moved from the cytoplasm into the mitochondria and help to trigger autophage.

Beta amyloid—a specific type of amyloid protein, composed of linear nonbranching fibers, formed into sheets and plaques, with hyperphosphorylation and forming an inflammatory reaction from astrocytes and microglia.

Bid—is a protein product which when transported into the mitochondria it helps trigger autophagy.

Bradykinesia—a decrease in spontaneity or movement.

Cannabinoids—organic substances present in Cannabis sativa, having a variety of pharmacological properties.

Cannabinoid receptors—also inhibit N—and Q-type calcium channel activity, which controls calcium entrance into the cells; they stimulate potassium (K+) channel conductance, allowing more potassium into the cells.

Cascade—a sequence of interactions, once initiated continues until completed, each interaction is activated by the preceding one.

Caspase 3—a protein that begins a cascade of enzymes that lead to cell apoptosis or cell death.

Chemokines—a chemical which is used to attract other cells.

Chemotactic—movement of cells in response to chemicals, or complement factors moving toward higher concentrations.

Cholinergic—nerve cells or fibers that use acetylcholine as their neurotransmitter.

Complement System—a group of heat-labile components in the serum, they can be destructive to certain bacteria and other sensitized cells which have been marked with complement-fixing antibody. C is a group of approximately 20 distinct serum proteins, these interact through enzymes and produce cleavage of cell membranes. They are designated from C1 through C9; subunits are designated by letters a, b, etc.

Complex II—a series of enzymes in the mitochondria that help convert food to energy.

Cryptic foci—abnormal areas within the colonic crypts, pitlike depressions in the colonic surface.

Dendritic cells—immune cells that process and present antigens to effector immune cells, located in lymph nodes.

Dopaminergic denervation of the striatum—when these cells no longer provide dopamine stimulation then the areas where these neurons affect they no longer have the dopamine stimulation, this greatly affects movement.

Dopaminergic neurons—nerve cells or fibers that use dopamine as their neurotransmitter.

Down-regulation—to reduce production, activity.

Eicosanoids—physiologically active substances derived from arachidonic acid.

Endothelial cells—flat cells which line blood vessels, lymphatic vessels and the heart.

Endotoxin—a bacterial toxin which is not released into the surrounding medium, it remains on the bacterial cell wall.

Eosinophils—a subtype of leukocytes, found in the blood and tissues, usually associated with allergies and parasitic infections.

Equilibrative nucleoside transporter 1—a protein that encodes for a membrane glycoprotein that transports nucleosides from the surrounding medium, found in cell and mitochondrial membranes.

ERK pathway—extracellular signal regulated kinase, when activated will lead to apoptosis or cell death.

Excitotoxicity—the process of exciting cells and then poisoning them; leads to nerve injury and death.

Exocytosis—the process of a cell excreting its secretory granules from inside the cel to the outside environment.

Extracellular Matrix—the components outside the cells that supports the cells.

Fibrillar species—referring to the non-digestable fibrils formed in Alzheimer's disease.

Fibroblast—a stellate or spindle shaped cell with cytoplasmic processes present in connective tissues, capable of forming collagen fibers.

GABAnergic neurons—gamma-aminobutyric acid, a calming or inhibitory neurotransmitter, stimulation of GABA reduces activity in the neurons.

Globulins—family of proteins that circulate in the blood, some are precursors to active compounds and others are immunoglobulins for protection, divided into alpha, beta and gamma.

Glucocorticoid—any steroid-like compound capable of influencing intermediary metabolism and of exerting an anti-inflammatory effect; cortisol is the most potent naturally occurring compound in our bodies.

Homolog's to retroviral oncogenes—our oncogene DNA segments are identical to retroviral oncogene and proto-oncogenes, the belief is that the retroviral genes were incorporated into our DNA.

HPA—hypothalamic-pituitary-adrenal axis—plays a pivotal role in our response to stress, preparing the body for fight or flight.

hyperesthesia—a condition with an abnormal increase to sensitivity of sensory stimuli.

hypoacetylation of H3 histones—the huntingtin protein in the abnormal form binds to the DNA and prevents some gene information from being transcribed, this is accomplished by reducing the acetylation of some H3 histonesbound to the chromatin.

Hypoxia-inducible transcription factor—when cells are living in reduced oxygen this transcription factor is activated to help the cells adapt to low oxygen, CBD prevents this protective process from occurring.

Intercalated nuclei—a cluster of neurons in the amygdala, when inhibitory tone is reduced there is an indirect reduction in anxiety by their effect on the central amygdala.

Intracytoplasmic inclusion bodies—a conglomeration of proteins which have accumulated inside the cell and cannot be removed or broken down.

Leukocytes—immune system cells, typically present in lymph tissue and the blood; there are 3 different types depending on their origin: myeloid, lymphoid and monocytic.

Ligand—a molecule that binds to a specific receptor.

Lymphocytes—white blood cells, derived from lymph tissue, circulate in the blood, two types. B and T, which are involved in our immune protection.

Macrophage—a monocytic cell which lives in the tissues, they function to engulf and take in inert substances and bacteria; participate in immune function through presentation of antigens to lymphocytes and secrete various immune modulatory compounds.

MAPK cascade—mitogen activated protein kinase—these are involved in helping the cell to respond to different stimuli or stressors, help regulate cell proliferation, gene expression, differentiation, mitosis, cell survival, and apoptosis.

Mast cells—mainly reside near small blood vessels, activation effects the permeability of blood vessels, activity increases with immune function.

Matrix Metalloproteinases—an enzyme that breaks down proteins, its action is dependent on incorporating a metal, zinc, or cobalt.

Mineralocorticoid—one of the steroids of the adrenal cortex that influence water and electrolyte (sodium and potassium ions) metabolism and balance.

Monocyte—a leukocyte with one large nucleus, circulates in the blood, spleen, lymph nodes, and loose connective tissue.

Monomeric—only having a single component.

mu-opioid receptors—one of three types of opioid receptors.

N-acetyl asparate—derived from the amino acid aspartate, which has been acetylated, second most common compound found in the brain.

Neoplastic—abnormal tissue that grows by cellular proliferation more rapidly than normal and continues to grow even after the initiating stimulus has ceased, structure and function is different from normal tissues and usually form a distinct mass.

Neural progenators—these are the stem cells which can produce neurons, or have the potential to become nerve cells.

Neurogenesis—formation of the nervous system, stimulating the production of neurons.

Neuromodulatory function—any compound that can affect the activity of the brain, as in changing the effects of neurotramsmitters (either their release or functional activity).

Neutrophilic—pertaining to neutrophils which are mature immune cell from the granulocytic series, also known as inflammatory cells.

Neutrophils—mature white blood cells, found in the blood and can move into tissues.

Nigrostriatal dopaminergic neurons—efferent neuron connections between the substantia nigra and the striatum, they use dopamine for their neurotransmitter.

Nitrosantive—to reduce a nitrosyl free radical.

Nitrosive stress—increased production of nitroysl free radicals.

Nitrosylated—a free radical formed from nitrogen and oxygen bonded togather.

NK cells—specialized immune cells that kill cancer cells and protect against intracellular infections by viruses, parasites and bacteria.

Nocioceptive—capable of appreciating or transmission of pain.

Oligodendrocytes—one of the three types of glial cells, the other two being astrocytes and microglia, along with neurons these cells make up the central nervous system; these produce the sheet-like processes which are wrapped around individual axons to form the myelin sheath; these protect the axon and speed up the neural transmission speeds.

Oligomeric—a compound with a few repeating units.

p38MAPK—mitogen activated protein kinase which is activated by cell stress and cytokines, they are involved in apoptosis (cell death) autophage self-destruction by the cell itself and cell differentiation.

Palmitoylethanolamide—another endocannabinoid which is derived from fatty acids, it participates in the entourage effect, does not bind to CB1 or CB2 receptors.

Paternal transmission—this is passed through the father's genes.

Pathogenesis—the pathologic, physiologic, or biochemical mechanism resulting in the development of a disease or morbid process.

Paw treading—rubbing pads of forelimbs, this is a sign of nausea which is seen in rats.

Phosphorylation—addition of a phosphate to an organic compound.

Phospholipids—a lipid containing phosphrous, including lecithins and other Phosphatidyl derivatives, the basic components of biological membranes.

Phytocannabinoids—plant derived cannabinoids, not synthetic.

PolyQ forms—aggregates of huntingtin protein, normally they are soluble and in Huntington's disease they are insoluble.

Present antigens—antigen presentation—some subtypes of immune cells will engulf the intruder and then process it; when this is complete the cell will then display the specific antigens to effector cells and then they will produce antibodies to attack the antigens on the invader cells; this can be accomplished through direct cell activity, antibodies which are released and by the complement system.

Protease—an enzyme that breaks down proteins/polypeptide chains.

Pyrogen—any agent that can cause fever.

Raf-1—also known as RAF proto-oncogene serine/threonine-protein kinase, proto-oncogene c-RAF, c-Raf it is part of the MAPK pathway, help regulate growth and cell division.

Retrograde diffusion—this moves in the opposite direction that nerve impulses are traveling, moving backwards across the synaptic cleft between two neurons.

S296 in the third transmembrane domain—this particular is a domain in glycine receptors in the spinal cord where CBD exerts some of the reduction in neuropathic pain, this reduces the nociceptive input for pain perception.

Senescence—the state of being old.

Somatodendritic—a particular site on the body of neurons in the substantia nigra pars compacta, these have neuromodulatory effects on nausea.

Striatum—collective name for the caudate nucleus, putamen and the globus pallidus.

Striatal atrophy—loss of neurons in the striatum.

Substantia nigra—a group of nerve cells in the brain stem.

Substantia nigra pars compacta—a group of nerve cells in the brain stem that use dopamine as their neurotransmitter and are involved in reward, addiction and movement.

Superoxide dismutase—an enzyme that converts 2 oxygens and 2 hydrogens into hydrogen peroxide and oxygen.

Synovial cells—cells which makeup the synovial membrane of a joint.

Tau protein—a protein that associates with microtubules and other elements of the cytoskeleton; found in the plaques of Alzheimer's disease.

THC—tetrahydrocannabinol, delta-9-tetrahydrocannabinol.

T-Helper 1—Th1 cells—a specific set of T lymphocytes that function in cell mediated immunity, these are CD8 lymphocytes and NK cells, these cells attack viruses, cancer cells and cells where invaders are inside and replicating, these are the cells that create chronic inflammation.

Thromboxanes—a group of compounds in the eicosinoids, related to prostiglandinws, they influence platelet aggregation, clot formation and an oxygen containing 6 member ring.

Transmembrane amyloid precursor proteins—proteins residing in a position through the cell membrane, these precursors can be converted into amyloid proteins; which cannot be dissolved by the enzymes.

Tumor Necrosis Factor-alpha—main cytokine for beginning and propagating an imflammatory response, activates immune cells and causes degranulation of other immune cells, causing the increase of inflammation.

Tyrosine hydroxylase—the enzyme that converts the amino acid l-tyrosine into L-DOPA.

Ubiquitin-proteasome system—a group of enzymes that provide protean breakdown for disposal.

Up-regulation—to increase production of molecules.

Vasoactive amines—influence the tone and caliber of blood vessels.

VCAM-1—this is an adhesion molecule which attracts and encourages more inflammatory cells to enter the area.

Vesicle—a closed structure surrounded by a single membrane.

About the Author

An international lecturer, author, and pediatrician, **Dr. John Hicks** has practiced integrative medicine for over thirty-five years. With an innovative approach to chronic disease, Dr. Hicks uses objective laboratory analysis to individualize medical and nutritional support, applying progressive and proven treatments to the physical and emotional well-being of each patient.

In recent years, Dr. Hicks has been recognized as an authority on medicinal cannabis and its application to a wide range of chronic illnesses and diseases. His focus has centered on the human endocannabinoid system and how cannabidiol—better known as CBD—provides powerful anti-inflammatory modulation, helping patients who suffer from dysfunction of their immune and nervous systems. He lectures around the country on medicinal marijuana, and specifically on the use of CBD.

Dr. Hicks graduated from the University of Louisville School of Medicine and spent two decades with a traditional pediatric practice in the Midwest before shifting his focus to holistic medicine. He is the author of numerous articles for a variety of health journals, including the *Autism Science Digest*, *Health Wise*, and others. Additionally, Dr. Hicks was a contributing author to the books *Cutting Edge Therapies for Autism* and *Bugs, Bowels, and Behaviors*.

Dr. Hicks lives in Los Gatos, CA with his wife and stepdaughter. He is the founder and medical director of Green Health Medical Group, a private practice focusing on holistic pediatric and family medicine. More information about his work can be found at www.johnhicksmd.com. For information on the practice, please visit, www.greenhealthmedicalgroup.com.